On the death of a child

On the death of a child

Celia Hindmarch

BA (Hons), Certificate in Counselling

RADCLIFFE MEDICAL PRESS●OXFORD and NEW YORK

©1993 Radcliffe Medical Press Ltd
15 Kings Meadow, Ferry Hinksey Road, Oxford OX2 0DP

Radcliffe Medical Press Inc
141 Fifth Avenue, Suite N, New York, NY 10010, USA

British Library Cataloguing in Publication Data

A catalogue record for this title is available from the British Library.

ISBN 1 870905 19 9

Typeset by Advance Typesetting Ltd, Oxfordshire
Printed and bound in Great Britain

Contents

About the author   vii
Acknowledgements   vii
Preface   ix

Introduction   xv

SECTION 1 Theory and Practice   1
1 Incidence and characteristics of child death   3
   The death of a child is different from other bereavements   3
   Sudden and accidental deaths   6
   Prenatal and perinatal loss   11
   Death from illness   15
   Death from congenital conditions   17
   Socially difficult deaths   19
   Reference   22

2 Features of grief and mourning when a child dies   23
   Bereavement theory   24
   Grieving for a child   30
   The concept of enduring grief   32
   So what is normal?   33
   Rituals   42
   References   44
   Further reading   45

SECTION 2 Good Practice Guidelines   47
3 Professional roles   49
   Ambulance personnel   49
   Clergy   51
   Funeral directors   52
   General practitioners   54
   Health visitors   56
   Hospital doctors   58
   Nurses   60
   Midwives   62
   Police   64

Registrars of births, marriages and deaths 66
Social workers 67
Teachers 69

4 Guidelines for all 71
General principles 71
Supervision 75
Training 77
Skills 78
Helping strategies 79
Resources questionnaire 81

5 Guidelines for stressful situations 83
Breaking bad news 83
Emergency procedures and intensive care 86
After the death 88
Attending the funeral 91
On first visiting the family 92
Anniversaries 94
Suicide risk assessment 94

SECTION 3 Support for Families 97
6 Bereavement support strategies 99
Practical support 99
Befriending 101
Counselling 102
Psychotherapy 106
Psychology 107
Psychiatry 107
Groups 108
Social activities 111
Support for children 112
Cultural differences 115
Further reading 115

7 Guidelines for support services 116
Core conditions 116
Starting a support group 117
A co-ordinated approach 120
The way forward 123
Further reading 124

Further reading 125

Useful addresses 127

Index 131

About the author

Celia Hindmarch is currently a freelance counsellor and trainer, and part-time tutor on counselling diploma and certificate courses at Manchester University and South Cheshire College. She was previously manager and senior counsellor at the Alder Centre bereavement support project, Liverpool.

Acknowledgements

The author is indebted to all those who have contributed directly and indirectly to the book, and in particular to those who have shared their personal experience of grief on the death of a child.

The writing of this book was made possible by the generosity of the **Duncan Norman Trust**, Liverpool, by awarding a grant to cover the author's research expenses.

All royalties from the sale of the book will go to the **Alder Centre** in recognition of their support.

Preface

The Alder Centre experience

The Alder Centre is situated at the Royal Liverpool Children's hospital at Alder Hey. Its remit is to support all those affected by the death of a child, of whatever age and from whatever cause. The Centre recognizes that the effects of a child's death extend far beyond the immediate family and includes all those involved in the care of the child and family before, during and after the death.

This pioneering project, initiated by a small group of health care professionals in partnership with bereaved parents, has become recognized as a model of good practice nationally and internationally. It evolved from the good work already being done by individuals and groups, and used their experience to form a vision of what more could be achieved by a multipurpose centre. The lessons learned so far form the basis of this book.

A brief history

In 1983 a small group of hospital social workers and nurses initiated an open meeting for all interested staff to review the hospital's approach to terminal care and bereavement follow-up support. This led to the formation of a group, which set itself the tasks of identifying good practice and creating new resources to supplement existing services. This Bereavement Core Group, as it came to be known, comprised highly motivated staff from a variety of disciplines and grades, and reflected a concern about the psychosocial context of health care.

The initiatives undertaken by the Group started with a survey of private space for families on the wards, which resulted in the designation of rooms in key areas for parents to be alone with their dead child. A comprehensive information booklet offering sympathy and practical advice to parents was produced. A questionnaire of staff needs led to training days for hospital workers, workshops for community health workers and input on training programmes for student nurses and doctors. Meanwhile, the social work department facilitated support groups for bereaved parents, who began exploring the idea of a drop-in centre.

In 1984 a crucial development took place with the introduction of parents to the Core Group. This signalled recognition of the importance of involving parents in the provision of care relevant to their needs. The philosophy of a partnership between parents and professionals grew from here. The presence of parents added a dimension of urgency and reality to the Group's work. The participation of parents in teaching sessions helped staff to gain confidence in the value of their efforts.

By 1987 plans were being formulated to make the vision of a drop-in centre into a reality, to supplement, co-ordinate and extend the support work already developed. It was a brave vision, and those who welcomed the opportunity to raise public awareness had to counter opposition from those who feared unwholesome publicity. However, hospital management proved sympathetic to the experiment, and made available a suite of rooms in the hospital grounds. The Bereavement Core Group re-formed as an Advisory Group to plan and launch the Alder Centre.

Setting up the Centre

Social Services backed the project by seconding a senior Alder Hey social worker part-time to co-ordinate the fund-raising, building altera-tions and refurbishment, publicity and administrative tasks. A clerical assistant was employed, who later became the Centre's first secretary. The Advisory Group, comprising parents, social workers, nursing and medical staff, met regularly to shape developments.

Philosophy

This was already clearly established – to operate the Centre as a partnership between parents and professionals in a non-medical setting and with open access.

Aims

The central aim, which became the Centre's remit, was defined as supporting anyone affected by the death of a child. The secondary aim was to raise awareness about the needs of bereaved families.

Objectives

It was expected that this support would take the form of individual counselling, groups, befriending and providing a place where people could come and feel a sense of belonging. More specific objectives included setting up a telephone helpline, hosting a Book of Remem-brance, providing a library, newsletter and information bank and addressing the needs of siblings. Raising awareness would involve training initiatives for professionals, developing links with other agencies and sensitive use of the media.

Premises

Much thought and care was given to decorating and furnishing the rooms in a way that provided a homely and comfortable atmosphere.

Staffing

Two full-time, trained counsellors were recruited to implement the Centre's services, supported by a full-time secretary. The senior counsellor was also designated as the manager, to oversee the day-to-day running of the Centre, with the Advisory Group in a supportive role. The counsellors were required to be able communicators and group facilitators, and were responsible for the training and support of 50 or so volunteers, mostly bereaved parents, to help run the Centre services. Parents were involved in the selection of staff.

Funding

The cost of equipping the Centre and running it for at least 2 years, employing three full-time staff, was estimated at £100 000. Liverpool Health Authority allocated £30 000 from cancer charity funds; another £30 000 was donated by the Nuffield Provincial Hospital Trust and large commercial organizations; and the remainder was found by the fund-raising efforts of parents and the generosity of the local community.

Publicity

Leaflets and posters were designed with a distinctive logo and disseminated widely at the time of the launch. Founder parents gave interviews for the media and articles were published in relevant professional journals.

The Centre was officially opened by the wife of Liverpool's Lord Lieutenant, herself a bereaved parent, at the end of June, 1989, three months after the Hillsborough Disaster.

The first year

The initial response to the opening threatened to overwhelm the staff with the number of queries and requests for help. The hard work of parents and goodwill of hospital staff maintained an ambitious programme and enabled the Centre staff to tick off the shopping list drawn up by the Advisory Group. An evening helpline opened, staffed by trained volunteers, and parents took responsibility for the monthly newsletter and library. The Centre's first Candle Service at Christmas was a moving and creative occasion. Support groups of different kinds evolved in response to current needs, including one for teenagers and one for grandparents, as well as the established groups for bereaved parents. Founder parents befriended new contacts, giving hope and reassurance for survival. Volunteers met at the Centre for training, support, fund raising and social meetings. Nurses on high-stress wards formed their own support groups. The Centre served as a focus for the various professionals around the hospital who were concerned with staff development, and a questionnaire revealed many requests for training as a means of support. This led to a Centre-co-ordinated training programme for hospital staff, which included counselling skills, stress management, self-awareness and aspects of bereavement. Student nurses visited the Centre as part of their training. Interested professionals from all over the UK and Europe attended monthly open days to learn about the Centre's work and to share their own experience.

Media attention provided welcome opportunities to raise awareness of the needs of bereaved families, although careful monitoring was needed to prevent sensationalism and exploitation. The BBC TV 40 Minutes documentary, *A Place for Tom*, which was screened in January 1990, gave a sensitive portrayal of the work of the Centre. The programme was a landmark in the Centre's development, putting it on the national map and inspiring a network of contacts with others seeking to improve local resources. The Readers' Digest commissioned Monica Dickens to write a feature, which was published in December 1990.

Requests for talks and conference workshops were met wherever possible with a joint input by Centre staff and founder parents. This was sometimes at considerable emotional cost to parents, but was always welcomed as a way of using their own experience to benefit others.

Achieving so much raised expectations of doing more. This seemed to reflect the common feature of parents feeling unable to do enough for the child who died, and the frustration of professionals feeling unable to 'help' the bereaved. Valid concerns focused on the capacity of the Centre to reach out to those sections of the community conspicuous by their absence, notably from the inner-city and ethnic minorities. An outreach worker was appointed with the brief to work in the community, to research and develop local resources, and specifically to liaise with the Hillsborough Project's work with bereaved families.

At the end of that first year, the data showed that half the referrals came directly from parents, and that the growing reputation of the Centre was attracting more contacts where the child died *suddenly* from all over Merseyside. These families emerged as the most vulnerable to isolation.

Developments

In the second and third years, growth and consolidation went hand in hand. A visit by the Princess of Wales provided further recognition of the Centre's purpose and value. The outreach worker initiated holidays for bereaved siblings to swim with Freddie the dolphin in the North Sea.

Another new development was the introduction of holiday breaks for families in the Lake District. An anthology of newsletter poems and prose was published, entitled *Enduring, sharing, loving* (Shawe, 1992). The Candle Service moved to Liverpool's Anglican cathedral to accommodate the growing numbers.

Social workers from the maternity hospital initiated groups at the Centre for neonatal loss and loss by miscarriage. Groups also ran for parents of older children, parents bereaved by accidental death and parents of murdered children. Informal social gatherings helped to integrate 'new' and 'old' parents. In the community, a room at the inner-city children's hospital was dedicated to the Centre's use, and the Centre assisted with setting up community support groups at Kirkby and on the Wirral.

The staff grew to six, with the arrival of the training co-ordinator to cope with growing demands for training, and later of the receptionist, to separate reception from administrative functions. External requests for training input came from teachers, occupational therapists and the police. At the hospital the Centre organized a study day for regional paediatricians and filled a regular spot on medical undergraduate courses. Internally, volunteers were eager for ongoing training, which would develop their individual and group skills.

Further afield, the Laura Centre opened in Leicester, modelled on the Alder Centre, and other hospitals visited to share their plans for starting similar projects.

Meanwhile, the hospital's new Trust status required a review of the Centre's relationship with the hospital management, the authority of the Advisory Group and long-term funding of the Centre. The outcome was the drawing up of a formal constitution for the Advisory Group and an undertaking by the hospital to absorb the core costs of the Centre – leaving the fund raisers free to fund developmental projects. The Centre had proved its worth, and was regarded as an ongoing resource.

The rapid growth of the Centre proved a constant challenge to balancing the needs and priorities of different groups of people who had an investment in its various activities. The task of ongoing evaluation, along with the assessment of research needs, was taken on by a small subgroup. The results of an evaluation questionnaire emphasized the importance of maintaining the homeliness of *A Place for Tom* alongside the work that gains professional credibility.

Some of the lessons learned from the Centre's first three years are included in the last chapter of this book.

Reference

Shawe M (Ed.) (1992) *Enduring, sharing, loving*. Darton, Longman & Todd, London.

Introduction

The authority for writing this book derives from the first years of the Alder Centre, a pioneering partnership between professionals and bereaved parents on Merseyside, co-ordinating support for bereaved families and their carers. The Preface outlines the story of this enterprise.

The observations and guidelines offered here are thus grounded in practical experience rather than drawn from academic research. The author is indebted to all those family members and professionals, from a range of disciplines, who have contributed to the learning embodied in this work. The learning has been gained by following the first guiding principle which is advocated for professionals offering support: *the importance of listening to what individual people say they want rather than presuming what they need.* The only experts are bereaved family members themselves. Their experiences are quoted to endorse the core messages that emerge: their need for understanding, information, choices and control.

Those whose work only rarely brings them into contact with child death will be unsure how to respond. What can they say or do that is helpful, or is at least not hurtful? It feels risky to come so close to such untimely loss and trauma. How will they cope? Are they qualified to help? Will they become anxious or depressed as a result of working with those bereaved of a child?

Those whose work brings them into regular contact with terminally ill children and bereaved families, even when that work becomes a chosen specialism, are never immune from such fears and apprehensions. Ways have to be found of coping with feelings of failure and helplessness, which avoid hard-nosed denial at one extreme, and compassion fatigue at the other. So this book is designed to inform those who are inexperienced in dealing with child death, to encourage those who are already familiar with the issues and to help both groups assess their own abilities and limitations. Guidelines can provide a useful checklist against experience and it is the author's hope that they will build confidence and reassurance. Underconfidence can lead to bereaved parents and siblings being referred on for specialist help that may not be appropriate nor available. It is the nature of grief that makes the front-line professional feel inadequate.

All aspects of child death are covered. Although case examples and statistics relate to the ages 0–19, it is recognized that the child status extends from prebirth to any age while parents are alive to grieve their loss. There are three sections: the first deals with definitions and context, and includes challenging the adequacy of conventional bereavement theory when applied to child death; the second offers guidelines related to the various roles and tasks, which may be undertaken by different individuals and professional support services; and the third section gives an overview of various support resources and strategies, leading to guidelines on the setting up of specific services.

Selected reading may be preferred according to interest and experience, but it is hoped that all readers will refer to the core messages contained in Chapter 4. These are simple but not always obvious. The most important ingredient in effective support is the relationship between helper and bereaved. Whatever the nature of that relationship, whether health professional/patient, teacher/student, social worker/ client, priest/parishioner, as friends or colleagues, common core conditions can be identified which help to create trust. Sensitivity cannot be taught, but awareness of the issues can be developed and skills can be practised. The need for adequate support and supervision is strongly argued as being fundamental to professional good practice in this specially stressful area of bereavement care.

Use of gender

For convenience, references are made to the dead child as male, and to the surviving sibling as female. At the risk of reinforcing stereotypes, adults are referred to in the predominant gender for the role or situation being considered.

SECTION 1
Theory and Practice

1 Incidence and characteristics of child death

Although this book covers many different situations involving the death of a child, all of them heartbreaking, it is important to remember that it is now a comparatively rare event in the Western world. Thankfully, most children recover from their accidents or illnesses nowadays. Modern health care and technology ensure that most childhood diseases can be cured or controlled.

But some children do die. In 1991, the deaths of children aged 0–19 in England and Wales totalled 12 235 (*see* Table 1.1) or 8986 excluding stillbirths (*see* Table 1.2). The impact of child death is out of all proportion to its incidence, in terms of the number of people affected and the severity of the effects. The factual data presented here are compiled from various sources, and are supported by the experiences of parents and staff of the Alder Centre in Liverpool, the first centre of its kind established to support those affected by the death of a child.

The death of a child is different from other bereavements

Those who have lost a parent, a spouse and a child will invariably describe their grief for the child as the most painful, enduring and difficult to survive. For emergency services personnel, the death of a child is the casualty they most dread having to deal with. For medical and nursing staff, there is a special sense of failure and frustration when a child dies.

The enduring pain of losing a child cannot be measured, so that it is not possible to say that it is more or less painful to lose a child suddenly or after a long, debilitating illness; nor can it be assumed that the age of the child determines the intensity of the emotions (*see* Figure 1.1). In terms of adjustment, parents of older children have the benefit of more positive memories to draw on, although in another sense they have more to lose, having built up a relationship with the child in its own right. Mixed groups at the Alder Centre have illustrated time and again

Table 1.1 Number of child deaths (age 0–19 years) by cause in England and Wales 1991

Category of death	Number	Percent
Sudden and accidental deaths	**3294**	**26.9**
sudden death, cause unknown (including SIDS)	919	7.5
road vehicle accidents	912	7.5
other accidents	1463	12.0
Perinatal deaths (excluding SIDS)	**6301**	**51.5**
stillbirth	3249	26.6
neonatal deaths	3052	24.9
Death from illness	**1409**	**11.5**
Death from congenital conditions and those arising at birth	**967**	**7.9**
Socially difficult deaths	**264**	**2.2**
suicide	128	1.0
murder	54	0.4
drug misuse	82	0.7
Total of major categories	**12 235**	**100.0**

Source: Office of Population Censuses and Surveys (1991) Mortality statistics. HMSO, London.

Table 1.2 Total number of child deaths from all causes in England and Wales 1991

Sex	Age (years)				
	Under 1	1–4	5–9	10–14	15–19
Male	2966	554	341	354	1208
Female	2192	439	248	222	462
Total	**5158**	**993**	**589**	**576**	**1670**

Source: Office of Population Censuses and Surveys (1991) Mortality statistics. HMSO, London.

the humility and generosity of one parent respecting another parent's experience, expressed here by Dave:

> When my son Paul was killed in a road accident, a week after starting his first job, I didn't see that I had anything in common with younger parents who had lost a baby. But when I have heard such parents talking in a group I recognize the same pain. I feel so sorry for those parents. At least we had our son for 19 years.

However, it is certainly a different experience, with different factors to be taken into account. The characteristics of various situations will be considered by grouping the deaths into five main categories according to cause and circumstance (*see also* Table 1.1 and Figure 1.2):

- sudden and accidental deaths
- prenatal and perinatal loss
- death from illness
- death from congenital conditions
- socially difficult deaths.

Figure 1.1: Child deaths (age 0–19 years) from any cause in England and Wales 1991 (excluding stillbirths)

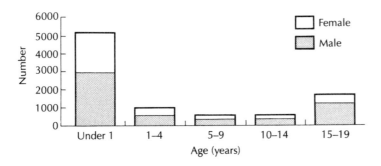

Source: Office of Population Censuses and Surveys (1991) Mortality statistics, HMSO, London.

Figure 1.2: Categories of death in children (age 0–19 years) in England and Wales 1991

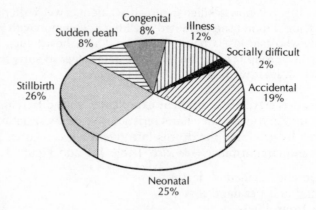

Source: Office of Population Censuses and Surveys (1991) Mortality statistics, HMSO, London.

Case studies are included to highlight certain characteristics, with the approval of the families concerned.

Sudden and accidental deaths

Cot death

'Cot death' is the generic term used to describe the sudden, unexpected death of an apparently healthy baby. In about one-third of these cases, the post-mortem discovers an adequate cause to explain the death, such as an overwhelming infection. For the remaining two-thirds, no cause of death can be found and the death is certified as *sudden infant death syndrome* (SIDS). In either case, no-one could have foreseen or prevented the death.

Extensive research has pointed to a number of tenuous coincidental factors for SIDS in both baby and environment, but these are not identified causes. The lack of explanation feeds the mythology associated with this tragic death: Ancient Sumerians believed the baby was stolen by evil spirits; the Bible records a woman's child dying in the night 'because she overlaid it' (1 Kings 3:19); some East European countries still routinely record unexplained infant deaths as infanticide.

Facts and figures

Incidence

Variations that occur in the figures for cot death in any given year depend on which definitions are used, the age range and on what appears on the death certificate. As an approximate guide, the incidence most commonly quoted for the UK has been two per 1000 live births, accounting for over 900 deaths in England and Wales in 1991 (*see* Table 1.1, page 4). However, there has been an encouraging drop in the rate in recent years, estimated at 35% from 1988 to 1991 by the Foundation for the Study of Infant Deaths. This has been linked to an extensive campaign to reduce the risk of cot death by identifying certain factors that may be *influential*, although not *causal* in themselves. The most significant of these relates to the sleep position, and the current advice is to place the baby on its back or side, to avoid overheating in babies who are unknowingly vulnerable. In the county of Avon, where the campaign has received its highest profile, the reduction in cot deaths over the last four years is reported to be a staggering 90% (50 deaths in 1988 down to four in 1992).

Age and circumstances

Cot death happens most frequently in the first six months of life, with a peak at two to three months. It is rare in the first month, and the rate drops sharply after six months to become increasingly uncommon in the second year of life. Babies who die suddenly and unexpectedly are typically found dead in their cots in the morning, but some die in the pram, the car, or even in their parents' arms. There are no symptoms, although some babies – perhaps coincidentally – will have had the 'snuffles' in the preceding days.

Males are more at risk than females, as are twins, preterm and low-weight babies. Cot deaths are twice as common in the winter months, peaking in December and January. They occur in all social classes, although there is a higher incidence among babies born to young mothers, mothers who have a short interpregnancy interval and those who do not present for antenatal care.

Legal procedures

A doctor has to confirm that the baby is dead, either at home or at hospital. As the death is sudden and unexpected, the doctor has by law to inform the coroner, or the procurator fiscal in Scotland. The coroner's officer, or more likely a police officer acting for the coroner, investigates the death by interviewing the parents. The CID may visit if a 999 call has been made. The baby's bedding and clothing are required to be seen and may be removed from the house. The baby is taken to the hospital by police, ambulance officer, doctor or funeral director, for a post-mortem examination to be carried out by a pathologist on the instructions of the coroner.

CASE STUDY

Tom was a bonny nine pound baby at birth. At seven months he developed a chest infection, which the GP treated with antibiotics. A week later, when Tom seemed fully recovered, the family woke one morning to find him still and lifeless in his cot. Tom's distraught parents, Dave and Sue, knew immediately he was dead, which was confirmed by their GP, who was first on the scene. After prescribing a sedative for Sue, he left with what seemed to the parents like undue haste. They later discovered that he had hurried home to check his seven-month-old baby girl before going to the surgery to look at Tom's notes to see whether he had missed something.

Meanwhile the police had arrived and completed their investigations with sensitivity. Most importantly for Sue, no-one tried to take Tom from her arms until she was ready to let him go. After a brief separation, while Sue and Dave followed Tom in the ambulance (although they wish now they had gone with him) they were reunited at the hospital.

> 'The staff were wonderful', Sue recalls 'A nurse brought Tom in to us holding him close, as if he was still alive, treating him with respect. It meant a lot to us that someone said how beautiful he was, and a couple of the staff sat and cried with us. There was no rush'.

They had to leave Tom for the post-mortem examination over the weekend, but were welcomed whenever they returned to hold him again. Tom was home for two days before the funeral, an important time for the parents and for Tom's six-year-old brother Graeme, who read his book of nursery rhymes to the baby as his way of saying goodbye. Dave and Sue thought it best that three-year-old Michael did not see Tom, but with hindsight now wish they had allowed this, as Michael suffered awful fantasies of what Tom looked like. Fortunately there were photographs to allay his fears.

Sue was left with the overwhelming guilt of knowing that Tom died as she and Dave were sleeping in the same room. 'It took over three years to accept that I couldn't have done anything – and I still find it difficult.'

Death by accident

A child is more likely to suffer accidental death than to die from an illness or abnormality (*see* Figure 1.2, page 6). A major cause of accidental death in children is road traffic accidents (RTAs), where the child may be a pedestrian or passenger, and in later adolescence may be the driver of the vehicle. Other accident situations include death by drowning, choking, burning, falling and poisoning. The death may be immediate or as a result of injuries, and the child's body is likely to be damaged externally, and sometimes severely maimed.

Whether or not other family members are involved in the accident, they will be suffering the effects of trauma. Extreme reactions of shock, disbelief and anger can be frightening and difficult for those in attendance.

Denial and evidence

Denial of what has happened is a natural defence and initially helps the traumatized system to cope. However, if the denial persists, the bereaved person will suffer from extreme anxiety and risks long-term mental health problems. Facing reality requires unambiguous explanation and evidence, and ultimately seeing is believing. The need to view the body or photographs of the deceased has been recorded by those who have worked with the relatives of disaster victims.

These were some of the conclusions reached by Janet Haddington after counselling families who lost a loved one in the sinking of the *Marchioness* in 1989 when, after the first two days, visual identifications of drowned relatives were first discouraged and then disallowed by the coroner's officers:

> The police should understand that identification may not be the sole reason for relatives wishing to view bodies. The bereaved also need to be clearly informed that photographs have been taken and will be made available at any stage in the future should seeing them feel helpful. The bereaved also need to be informed that once the body is released to the funeral director they have the right to view. The manner in which some bereaved have been denied access to view the body has led to long-lasting anger and protracted grief.

The use of the word 'denied' here is interesting, suggesting that professionals may seek to protect others from pain as a way of denying their own. Sometimes the mother is excluded from seeing the body in the belief that she is not strong enough to cope and may become hysterical.

Legal proceedings

The difficulty of dealing with intense grief reactions is exacerbated by legal proceedings, which may take months or even years to complete. The results of the post-mortem examination may be withheld when parents are anxious to learn every detail about injuries. Accidental death requires a coroner's inquest to establish the cause of death. Where a person has been charged with murder, manslaughter, causing death by reckless driving or infanticide, the inquest is adjourned until the conclusion of the criminal proceedings. The evidence of witnesses and the results of police investigations will not be known until then, leaving parents in an anguish of uncertainty. It helps if the police keep them informed and if the coroner prepares them for the inquest, but too often they feel doubly victimized by an adversarial legal system that excludes them. In the case of a road traffic accident death that leads to a criminal charge and trial, parents desperately want the offender to admit responsibility and show regret. Sadly, the inevitable process of prosecution and defence makes this almost impossible. Most parents seek reparation, not retribution.

However, sentences for convictions of careless, reckless or dangerous driving leave the family and community feeling that a child's life is held cheap. The same applies to amounts paid as compensation.

CASE STUDY

Seventeen-year-old Kevin was a cheerful and popular lad with a sense of fun and adventure. While waiting for the train home one Saturday night, Kevin and his mates explored the goods area of the station and climbed on top of a wagon. Kevin touched the overhead electric wires and was killed outright.

Kevin's mother Betty was called home from her night-shift by the news that Kevin had been involved in an accident. Fearing the worst, she arrived home to find that her husband Kenny had already been taken away by the police. Her telephone enquiries to the local hospitals and police stations all drew a blank, and she was left in an agony of not knowing what had happened. Meanwhile, at the railway station, Kenny was told by the British Transport Police how Kevin had died, and was advised not to see his body. The officer who gave this advice had not seen Kevin himself, but assumed the body to be badly burned. Kenny identified Kevin from his watch and ring.

Back home, Betty's fears were confirmed when one of Kevin's friends who had witnessed the accident returned to his home a few doors away. She was angry and distressed to be separated from Kenny at the time they most needed to be together.

On his return, Kenny told Betty what he knew, and they comforted each other and their daughters as best they could. They struggled with dreadful fantasies of what Kevin looked like and were anxious to know exactly what had happened. Two days after the accident they were shocked to read a tabloid newspaper report of the tragedy prefaced by the headline 'Fried Alive . . .'. They were upset to read that British Rail were concerned about the boys trespassing.

Before the funeral, the undertaker heard the tentative note in the parents' question: 'Would you advise us to see him?' He replied that it was up to them, but they might prefer to remember Kevin as he was. They were frightened to do otherwise than heed his advice. Consequently they did not know what they were burying: later, Kenny owned his vision of 'a burnt head of a matchstick'. Betty simply could not believe Kevin was dead. It had all been a ghastly mistake and one day he would just turn up at the back door, having been away on one of his army courses.

At the same time, Betty was inconsolable. She began to resent Kevin's friends and was convinced they were hiding the true story from her. She was advised not to go to the inquest, some four months later, as being 'too upsetting' for her. Kenny attended, and watched helplessly as photographs of Kevin's dead body were passed among the jury – photographs that he did not know existed.

Over three years later, Betty was still angry and bitter. 'I'm left with this void. If I had seen him, I would have known he was dead, instead of waiting for him to come home, which is what I still do.'

Disaster

The deaths of children caught up in a disaster, as at Aberfan, Hillsborough and Lockerbie, awaken themes of violence and senseless-ness. Where there are many deaths together, the intensity of the shared grief is overwhelming, and extremely difficult to resolve. This is com-pounded by the protracted legal battles to determine responsibility, and it is bitterly resented when no-one is held accountable. Fears of litiga-tion, compensation awards and individual job dismissal make it almost impossible for anyone to show the regret and remorse the parents badly want to hear expressed.

Prenatal and perinatal loss

Miscarriage

Miscarriage is also known as spontaneous abortion. Nobody knows the true incidence, as many early miscarriages are not reported, but it is estimated that over 20% of all clinically confirmed pregnancies end in miscarriage before 20 weeks' gestation. Allowing for the reality that some women feel relieved to miscarry in the event of an unwanted pregnancy, miscarriage still accounts for the highest incidence of child loss. After the age of viability, set at 24 weeks gestation in the UK, the fetus is regarded as a baby and its death described as a stillbirth. But for most parents, and particularly for the mother, the growing mass of cells has always been a baby. With the aid of ultrasound scans, parents can now see the growing shape and movements of their baby long before the mother can feel it move inside her.

Early miscarriage means there is nothing to say goodbye to, and no ritual to help make the loss a reality. Anguish and guilt may derive from not knowing what happened to the fetus, which becomes hospital property. Fortunately, growing awareness has enabled health professionals to acknowledge these anxieties. Mothers are now encouraged to see and hold a formed baby, however small, and many chaplains will arrange some kind of funeral long before the law requires it. Most parents will appreciate a scan picture, if one is available, as evidence that their baby existed.

Late miscarriage means the baby has died nearer to a viable age, redefined by the Stillbirth (Definition) Act 1992 as 24 weeks' gestation, and is legally entitled to a funeral. Medical terms such as 'placental insufficiency' and 'cervical incompetence' encourage the mother's feeling that she is to blame. The later the loss, the greater the attachment will have been between mother and baby, and to a lesser extent between father and baby, so that grief reactions are likely to be more intense. The importance of naming the baby, spending time to say goodbye, and a proper and dignified ritual, have all been established as helpful for healthy grieving. Photographs are usually treasured by the parents, and are helpful to other family members such as grandparents and siblings who were not able to see the baby.

CASE STUDY

Faye and Denis always planned to have two children. They hoped for a girl and a boy. Eighteen months after having Michael, Faye lost her second baby, Deborah, at 20 weeks:

> 'I was sure she had been dead for a couple of weeks, but at first no-one seemed to take me seriously when I said I knew something was wrong. I didn't even see her, and felt guilty afterwards. I didn't like to ask what happened to her little body, but I guessed. When I went back on the ward nobody knew what to say to me and I couldn't wait to get home.'

Having been told that she might not be able to carry another baby to term, Faye was apprehensive when she became pregnant again eight years later. She lost Jane at 17 weeks, but this was a very different experience.

> 'Denis came with me for the scan, which confirmed the worst, and he stayed with me when they induced labour. Jane was so tiny she could fit in your hand. We held her and had some photographs taken and the sister asked if we wanted the chaplain to come. We knew she couldn't baptize her but she did a sort of blessing, which meant a lot to us. Jane even had a proper little funeral service, and we can visit the Petal Garden at the local crematorium where the ashes of all premature babies are scattered. I just wish we could have done the same for Deborah.'

Termination

In 1991 the total number of recorded pregnancy terminations in the UK was 167 300. SATFA (Support After Termination For Abnormality) estimate that over 2000 of these terminations were advised or sought because of fetal abnormality.

Requested termination

Termination as a solution to unwanted pregnancy may be sought for a variety of reasons. In the younger age group, a girl's pregnancy may be at odds with her maturational and educational needs, it may be the result of forced sex or it may be the consequence of trying to get psychological needs met. For an older woman, there may be a conflict with other priorities at that time. She may fear that this baby will impose emotional, mental or physical demands that will be damaging to herself or her family. At any age, she may want the baby but is under pressure from family or partner not to continue with the pregnancy, and may lack the support she needs. Whatever the circumstances, termination is likely to be a negative choice with some level of regret. It may be necessary to deny this conflict of feelings in order to go through with the decision. The medical assessment that follows a request for termination subjects the woman to the kind of scrutiny that is not required of a woman who decides to have a child. Pre-abortion counselling is unlikely to uncover ambivalence or regret in women who do not feel able to make free choices.

Medically advised termination

If there is evidence that a baby will be born with a significant abnormality, either because of a congenital condition or because the baby has been exposed to potential damage, or if the continued pregnancy puts the mother's health at serious risk, then a termination will be offered to the mother. If she decides to terminate on the basis of uncertain risks, she may never know whether the baby would have been all right, and the responsibility of making such a painful decision will weigh heavily. Even when the choice is obvious, the mother is likely to feel guilt and a sense of failure. Again, these feelings may need to be denied at the time in favour of logic and common sense.

The termination of an abnormal fetus is experienced as a double bereavement, compounded by feelings of guilt and inadequacy that the baby was 'faulty'.

Stillbirth

In 1991, 3249 stillbirths were registered in England and Wales (*see* Figure 1.1, page 5). This figure will rise when the statistics from 1992 become available, as the Stillbirth (Definition) Act 1992 lowered the definition age for stillbirth from 28 to 24 weeks' gestation. There can be few more poignant and distressing experiences than to give birth to a dead baby, or be witness to this cruel loss. The stillness of a new-born baby is a tragic juxtaposition of life and death.

Stillbirths are registered as births and not as deaths. A separate stillbirth form records confidential information that is used only for the preparation of statistics by the registrar general. In the unusual case of a full inquest, a coroner's conclusion will be provided, but is not classified as a verdict because a stillborn baby is deemed not to have lived and therefore there has been no legal death. However, the registration provides an opportunity for confronting the reality and, as such, is a kind of ritual. Parents are issued with a certificate of registration. The Stillbirth and Neonatal Death Society (SANDS) has done much to raise awareness about the need of parents to say goodbye to their baby, and many hospitals now have a room or suite available away from the maternity ward.

Neonatal death

Neonatal means newly-born, and defines the period from birth to 28 days. This overlaps with the term 'perinatal', which applies to the period between the viability time of gestation (24 weeks) and the first seven days after birth, so for that first week the two words can be used synonymously. There were 3052 neonatal deaths in England and Wales in 1991 (see Table 1.1, page 4). The causes of neonatal death are common to stillbirth: abnormal development, premature delivery and complications during labour. The baby may have been born without the necessary capacity for survival, which is usually anticipated before the birth, or unexpected problems during the birth process damage an otherwise healthy baby. In the latter case the mother may be heavily sedated, have undergone an emergency caesarean section, and be quite unwell after the birth. Her own incapacity can have important consequences if the baby dies before she can relate to him.

The baby's initial attachments, however, are to machines and tubes, and the parents' first sight of their baby surrounded by technology and protected by a wall of plastic can be frightening. There is usually an intense longing to hold the baby, which may be frustrated until the baby dies. Neonatal Unit staff encourage parents to handle the baby whenever possible, and share the baby's care. However, it is common for parents to withdraw emotionally and physically from the baby in anticipation of their loss. This can be a source of acute feelings of guilt later on, and is distressing to the staff and other parents on the unit. The loss of a twin, when emotional energies are split between the surviving twin and the dying twin, is specially poignant.

The parents have experienced their baby as having an independent life. That life is valued, however short, and parents will specify hours and minutes when describing their loss. There is often a tragic sense of helplessness, for both parents and staff, as the fight for life is lost. The primary nurse, the consultant and the chaplain may assume great significance for the parents, as being the main characters in the baby's short life.

Death from illness

Malignant disease

The diagnosis of childhood cancer is not the death sentence it is often presumed to be, and around 70% of children with the most common form of leukaemia have a good prognosis of long-term survival. Treatments and therapies for cancers and blood disorders are often painful and distressing, involving disfiguring side-effects such as hair loss from chemotherapy and puffy weight gain from steroids. Periods of remission give rise to hope and optimism, but as successive treatments fail for those with a poor prognosis, there is time to prepare for the inevitable outcome.

Some parents and families do plan accordingly, and provide many varied life-experiences for their child's remaining months or years, such as trips abroad and visits to Disneyland. Others do not or cannot even talk about the future and cope by maintaining denial to the end. In either case the question remains whether it is ever possible to feel prepared for the reality of the death when it occurs. Stories are legion of the courage of these children in approaching death. The home services provided by specialist Macmillan nurses and Malcolm Sargent social workers can help to normalize the family's life and facilitate the child's death at home wherever possible.

CASE STUDY

David was 15 months old when his parents were told the diagnosis to explain a persistent lump (and his mother's intuition) that he was seriously unwell: a stage four neuroblastoma, with a very poor prognosis for recovery. Sue and John remember the compassion of the consultant at their local hospital who was clearly upset to tell them this bad news. David was transferred to the nearest paediatric hospital, Alder Hey in Liverpool, for the specialist treatment he needed. This was one of the worst times: arriving at a strange place at the weekend, when the ward was eerily quiet, and suddenly feeling totally out of control, shocked and angry that this was happening to their child.

Sue's philosophy is to face things head-on, and John's recent experience of losing both parents in an atmosphere of secrecy and denial made them both determined to be open about David's illness. They appreciated the Alder Hey consultant answering their questions honestly, balancing hope with realism. They came to feel part of a team, working together with medical and nursing staff, social worker and play therapist, and became part of a ward culture that enabled parents to support each other.

There followed a regime of chemotherapy, to which David responded well, with a week in hospital and two weeks at home. Sue and John readily responded to the Malcolm Sargent social worker's advice to include Jane, their three-year-old daughter, in what was going on. As a result, all three of them would sometimes stay with David on the ward at weekends. Otherwise Sue and John took it in turns to be with him while the other maintained a secure base for Jane. Throughout his illness, David's quality of life was high, and they were able to function as a normal family for much of the time. After six months, the time was judged right for surgery to remove the primary tumour. The immediate improvement in David's condition after the operation gave new hope – only to be dashed within weeks when tests confirmed that the cancerous growth had returned. This was the darkest hour for Sue and John, with the realization that time was running out. After David reacted badly to one last-chance experimental treatment, they felt he had had enough, and active treatment was stopped.

David died at home, without pain, two weeks before his second birthday, hours after watching his favourite Postman Pat videos together with his family. Sue describes it as an extraordinarily peaceful day.

Acute illness

Viral infections such as meningitis can overwhelm a child very quickly. By the time the parents become alarmed by symptoms and call the doctor or take the child to hospital, the child's condition is likely to have worsened rapidly. When the child dies, perhaps within a day or two, the loss is experienced as a sudden death, and the parents are caught in a nightmare of disbelief. Typically parents will blame themselves for not alerting the doctor earlier and so, maybe, reducing the chances of recovery. The mysterious power of an invisible killer disease that can strike without warning lends itself to quite irrational conclusions: parents may become convinced that a playmate was carrying the infection, or that a recent visit to the shops was somehow connected. Fears for the safety of surviving children are likely to run high and lead to overprotective attitudes. The family too may suffer from others' irrational beliefs that it is somehow contaminated by such tragic fortune and thus better avoided.

Death from congenital conditions

Cystic fibrosis

This is the most common genetically inherited life-threatening disorder. Diagnosis follows recurrent chest infections in infancy, although the life-expectancy has increased steadily as symptom treatment has improved; many children with cystic fibrosis now survive into adulthood. Careful exercise and management can sustain a near-normal lifestyle for much of the time.

As the children and parents are in and out of hospital over a number of years, strong attachments form with hospital staff. Hospital and community nurses become part of an extended family, and they come to see the family as friends more than patients. Children who want to talk about their condition may protect their parents from distress by talking to a trusted nurse – perhaps at night when the child is alone and has time to think. The staff are therefore closely involved in the child's life and death.

Heart deformities

Over one-third of hospital child deaths relate to congenital heart conditions, although in a few cases the heart deformity develops as the result of a viral infection. In a large paediatric hospital, this amounts to an average of one or two deaths per week. Six children per 1000 are born with some kind of heart abnormality: of these, one-third die soon after birth, and one-third will require surgery. Although the child has had a chronically sick condition, the death is usually experienced as sudden, as most typically occurring in surgery and at a young age.

Although the parents are told the risks of survival, the faith required to hand over their child to the surgeon suspends any realistic view. The shock, disbelief and anger that parents experience are compounded by the fatal operation taking place when the child was in the best of health, to optimize the chances of coming through. Thus the parents may have brought in a comparatively healthy child who was skipping down the ward one day, and is dead the next.

One important consequence of this pattern of events is the guilt that parents feel that they were not with their child when he died, and the heavy sense of responsibility that, in consenting to this operation, they virtually signed a death warrant. Anger towards the surgeon and the hospital is often extreme, and more parents are resorting to litigation.

CASE STUDY

New-born baby Clare's feeding difficulties and a blueness around the lips alerted maternity staff that something was badly wrong. John and Maureen, her parents, were told there was a slim chance of her surviving the necessary surgery to insert a shunt. But she did survive, and came through major surgery at 18 months with flying colours. John remembers that they were totally oblivious to the risks at that time – perhaps because they didn't want to know – and had absolute faith in the surgeon.

To all outward appearances Clare grew up a very normal little girl: she went to a normal school, joined the Brownies, Guides and majorettes, and John taught her to swim. But she couldn't run about like other children, and her parents always had to be extra vigilant to make sure she didn't overdo things. And as she got older, the need for more corrective surgery grew with her. 'It was rather like living with a gas leak', John recalls. 'You don't realize the danger until someone comes in from outside and brings it to your notice. We didn't see how much Clare had deteriorated'.

It wasn't until the last year of Clare's life that John and Maureen realized that she might die. Meeting other parents through the Association for Children with Heart Disorders opened their eyes. With no other options left, Clare faced major surgery again at the age of ten and a half years, and this time she did not come through.

'Something inside me just knew she wouldn't make it', says John. 'We really started grieving for her from the time we were told of the operation – like picking up a newspaper dated three months later. But it was still an enormous shock to lose her'.

Neurodegenerative disorders

There are literally hundreds of genetically inherited life-threatening diseases, some very rare, which are mostly metabolic in origin. The most common of these conditions include the dystrophies and Batten's disease. The principle feature of these neurodegenerative disorders is the progressive deterioration of the neurological system over weeks, months or years. This often includes a distressing deterioration of mental faculty.

The timing of the diagnosis varies, but typically an apparently well child will develop non-specific symptoms such as epileptic fits, a squint or an awkward gait. At first the degeneration may be slow, and parents can suffer years of struggle and worry, perhaps being labelled as overanxious by the medical profession. As the symptoms increase and the condition worsens, tests lead to a diagnosis. The label makes no difference to the outcome, and the parents will be told that the condition is life-threatening. The bereavement starts here, and some anticipatory grieving will begin as the child's functioning becomes progressively worse.

Parents are desperate to know the prognosis, and most will ask: 'How long has he got?' Time limits and future plans become all-consuming pre-occupations. No-one can give a confident prediction of life expectancy, as the progression of the disease can remain on a plateau for several years. Care of the increasingly disabled child becomes the focus of family life, and respite care provides both a lifeline and a potential source of guilt for parents who become physically and emotionally exhausted.

Many of these children die in their early teenage years, usually from an infection which the debilitated system is unable to resist.

After such a death families are vulnerable to wounding remarks such as 'all for the best' and 'blessing in disguise'. Parents lose a lifestyle of care and a social network as well as their beloved child.

Socially difficult deaths

Some deaths carry an element of social stigma, presenting an added difficulty for families coming to terms with their grief. Murder, suicide, deaths associated with anorexia, substance misuse, AIDS, neglect and abuse evoke highly emotive responses at a social level. Such deaths are difficult to talk about, subject to myth and misunderstanding, and reduce the level of sympathetic support forthcoming in other situations. Bereaved families are thus likely to be further isolated.

Murder

The wounds may never heal for parents of murder victims. There may be an agonizing period of uncertainty between the discovery that the child is missing and finding the body, then again before the perpetrator is apprehended. If the body is not found, or is mutilated beyond recognition, the reality of the death is hard to reconcile. The legal process then takes over in a way that leaves the family feeling doubly victimized. Sensitive police handling of the case will take into account the importance of the family being kept as fully informed as possible. The parents are tormented by imaginings of their child's final violation, and their private grief is likely to be invaded by the media.

Suicide

Suicide is perhaps the biggest taboo of all, particularly in adolescence. It is hard to accept that a youngster, with all of life's potential before him, should choose to end it; suicide is a massive rejection of the parents who conceived and nurtured that life. The act of self-destruction, whether or not it was intended to result in death, may well happen at a time when family relationships are fraught and ambivalent.

Denial is an understandable defence against the burden of guilt and sense of failure that threaten to overwhelm the parents. Coroners often collude with this and return an open verdict if at all possible in order to spare the family's feelings. In fact, the uncertainty that follows an open verdict may hinder the grieving. As long as the parents can harbour the belief that there may have been a third party involved, or that an experiment went dreadfully wrong, they will engage all their energies in exploiting every theory that avoids facing reality.

In any case, the experience of social isolation is likely to be the same, adding a sense of shame to the guilt and responsibility. The stresses on parents and siblings are enormous, and suicidal thoughts of joining the dead youngster are commonly experienced. The expression of such dark feelings brings some relief, and contact with other families who have been through this ordeal can be reassuring.

Schools and colleges find it very difficult to deal with the suicide of a student. The events are usually shrouded in mystery and rumour, and a fear of copy-cat actions often prevents the staff from acknowledging the death openly. The myth that talking about suicide encourages others to feel suicidal still persists, while the healthiest outcome is for youngsters to express their feelings of shock and fear.

CASE STUDY

During the last three months of his life Simon had lost his job and written off his first car. In spite of these setbacks he did not appear to be depressed, and his family had no hint beforehand of his suicidal feelings. On a bitterly cold winter day he waited until his mother went out with the dogs, left a note for his parents, took some rope from the loft and made his way to a park behind a nearby pub. There he hanged himself from a tree in an area where he used to play as a child.

By the time the note was found and the police called, Simon's body had been discovered and taken to hospital. At first the police said there was still hope of the paramedics reviving him, when they knew he was dead, which later caused much resentment from the family. There was an agonizing two-hour wait before Simon's parents and two older sisters were allowed to go to the hospital. The police were perceived as kind but when they attempted to talk to Simon's father on his own Simon's mother felt hurt and demanded not to be left out. The family needed to be together and travelled to the hospital in the same car.

At the hospital the doctor who confirmed the death was experienced but cold and detached, and the family wished he had shown some feeling. The family found the nurses to be kind and considerate, and they were given as much time as they wanted with the body. Simon's older sister remembers being upset that his feet were not covered by the sheet.

Waiting for the inquest was a harrowing time, even though the suicide note left no doubt of the verdict. It read: 'Mum and Dad, I did something stupid today. So it is obvious my brain is not right or that I am not right. So I have gone to cure it for good. I love you very much, Simon.' Without any other explanation, the perplexed parents were deeply hurt by unfounded rumours that Simon had been thrown out of home, that he was on drugs, that he had 'got a girl into trouble'. They felt isolated by the implications that his home and family had been inadequate.

Substance misuse

Experimental use of drugs and other substances is widespread amongst young people, and in the UK almost universal as far as alcohol is concerned. The highest risk of accidental death occurs early on in the usage, when youngsters have low tolerance levels and are ignorant about the potentially lethal effects. Of the 82 deaths from drug misuse recorded in England and Wales in 1991 (*see* Table 1.1, page 4), it is believed that about one-third died on their first experience. Ambivalent and somewhat hypocritical social attitudes toward drug-taking do not help. Drugs education programmes that aim to minimize risk by giving children the information they need to stay safe are not promoted, on the grounds that such information encourages substance misuse. Parents may find it very difficult to come to terms with their child's behaviour, which was concealed from them, and seek scapegoats to blame. Often the family gets labelled as somehow inadequate.

AIDS

The HIV virus, which leads to this fatal syndrome, is communicated via body fluids, notably blood or semen. In the UK haemophiliac children have died and are dying as the result of receiving contaminated blood products from the USA in 1985–6. Obviously a particular feature of these deaths is the anger directed at the hospital for providing the contaminated blood. Alongside the anger is the guilt of parents who may have administered the fatal Factor VIII injection themselves. Increasingly, the incidence of AIDS in children is related to those born to HIV-infected mothers. It is not yet known what percentage of babies will remain infected after birth and how many will survive.

Such is the stigma attached to AIDS that most parents of these children are unable to share with others the true nature of their child's condition or cause of death. Some hospitals compound the stigma by isolating their HIV-positive patients. Sadly the experience of many parents indicates a reluctance by headteachers and governors to accommodate these children in their schools. Against this background, it is all-important for key professionals to encourage openness between children and parents as the disease progresses.

Care issues and fostering

Deaths that are linked in some way to neglect of the child or to non-accidental injuries evoke strong emotions. They usually take place against a background of deprivation and inadequacy. If the child dies with some real degree of parental responsibility, the parents' grief is likely to be ignored by a society that condemns them. The support of other bereaved parents is not available to them, and expert psychiatric care may be indicated.

Other issues arise with the death of a child who is not in the care of the birth parents. Foster-parents may be excluded from funeral arrangements made by the birth family. The death of a baby born to a girl who is herself in care will have implications for her carers too.

Reference

Haddington J (1992) Has it really happened? *National Association of Bereavement Services Newsletter*, 8, 1–5.

2 Features of grief and mourning when a child dies

'When my grandson died, some people thought I shouldn't be grieving the way I was. One person said that losing a child was no different to losing a much-loved partner or parent. I told her that if she ever lost a child or grandchild, to come back and tell me what she thinks then.'

'Don't talk to me about the grieving process . . . What a ludicrously inappropriate phrase to define the mental, physical and emotional turmoil you are left to sort out after your child has died.'

Both the grandmother and mother quoted here are expressing their frustration with the way society underestimates their experience of loss. They are saying that the death of a child *is* different from other bereavements, that this difference sets them apart from other people and that bereavement jargon is inadequate to describe the uniqueness of their experience and nature of their grief.

For professionals, too, there are special implications of dealing with the death of a child:

'I have had 20 years' experience as an accident and emergency nurse, and I can remember every child we've worked on and lost. I'm never prepared for that. I'm always drained afterwards, emotionally and psychologically. I just want to go home.

'I've been with the ambulance service over 13 years. Dealing with a child is totally different to an adult, and for me, cot death is more traumatic than anything else. I feel sick and totally useless.'

Whether personally or professionally involved, the death of a child is seen as the most difficult loss to cope with. It is also seen as the most difficult death to talk about and anticipate. It is important to acknowledge why this is so.

What does the death of a child mean?

Symbolically a baby represents the beginning of life and the ultimate in human creativity. A child symbolizes innocence, vulnerability, pleasure and potential for growth. Every adult carries some sense of the 'inner child' as a means of expressing the emotional and imaginative part of the psyche. At a deep psychological level, then, the death of any child violates that precious and vulnerable part of us. There is also a collective responsibility for children in society, and a corresponding investment in succeeding generations to carry forward present achievements and future aspirations. When any child dies, against the natural order of things, an important thread of continuity is broken.

Grandparents have an acute sense of this broken thread in the fabric of their own family as well as grieving the loss of the individual child.

Parents suffer multiple losses when their child dies. Obviously the primary loss relates to the attachment and dependency of a unique individual, while the absence of the child represents much more. Parents will also be grieving for other losses:

- part of their own sense of self, physically, emotionally and spiritually
- their connection to the future
- unfulfilled expectations and ambitions
- some of their own treasured qualities and talents
- a source of love and acceptance
- a sense of power and control over what happens to them
- social status and social contacts.

Siblings are often affected as much by their parents' grief as by their own. They also lose a sense of security in the world and are faced prematurely with their own mortality.

Carers' experience of loss will depend largely on their community or professional roles and level of involvement. The loss of faith in the power to help or heal is stressful. Those whose work commonly exposes them to a child death may lose all sense of normality.

More detailed consideration of how each of these groups is affected by the loss of a child will be given later in this chapter. First, it is necessary to look at bereavement theory in general to give a baseline understanding of grief reactions. The experience of bereaved parents and others will then be called upon to challenge the adequacy of general bereavement theory when applied to the death of a child. Religious and cultural differences will be taken into account whenever it seems relevant to do so.

Bereavement theory

Bereavement has come to mean the loss by death of someone close, although it originally referred to the marauding practices of bands of reavers many centuries ago, raiding the livestock of neighbouring clans. Thus, to be bereaved implies being robbed of deprived of something or someone of value, so that one is necessarily poorer for the loss.

This is a helpful concept for understanding the nature of grief. To be deprived of someone of value implies attachment, and the degree of attachment will determine the degree of loss experienced, which leads to grief:

- *bereavement* is what happens
- *grief* is what one feels in reaction to the bereavement
- *mourning* is what ones does to express grief.

Attachment bonds are formed from infancy to satisfy a basic need for security. The British psychiatrist John Bowlby, who did much to enlighten our understanding of attachment and loss, said that the important focus for understanding grief is what happens when attachments are threatened or broken: strong emotional reactions occur automatically (Bowlby, 1991).

When faced with loss, attachment behaviour is activated. This is readily observable at times when a mother is separated from her baby. The baby is distressed, cries and tries to cling to the mother to prevent her going; at the point of separation the baby protests angrily to get her back. If she returns, the baby's distress is alleviated; if not, the baby withdraws into apathy and despair.

This forms the pattern of the grieving process. These behaviours are geared towards retrieving the loss, and are repeated throughout life whenever one's sense of security is threatened. The automatic chain reaction of distress, anger and withdrawal follows the loss of a wallet and the death of a loved one.

The features of grieving

The features of grieving are well-documented and variously described to give some understandable pattern to grief reactions. This can be reassuring to those who are grieving, perhaps for the first time, and are overwhelmed by the extremes of feeling and behaviour they are experiencing. The idea of a shared road, which many have trod before, is comforting. The other main advantage of defined grief patterns is that the carer or professional supporting the bereaved has some kind of reference map for guidance.

On the other hand, describing grief as a process with different stages is fraught with difficulty. Human feelings cannot be parcelled up with neat labels and put into compartments. Bereavement is a complicated business, and is a unique experience. Few agree just how many stages there are supposed to be: some have listed as many as twelve! Colin Murray Parkes, the British psychiatrist whose research and writing on bereavement has been so influential, prefers the concept of phases, and describes four phases of mourning (Parkes, 1972). The American psychologist J William Worden, whose book *Grief counselling and grief therapy* is widely regarded as a standard text, adds the concept of tasks

Table 2.1 The four phases of grief

Phase	Features	Task
1. Denial	Shock, disbelief, sense of unreality	To accept the reality of the loss
2. Pain/distress	Hurt, anger, guilt, worthlessness, searching	To experience the pain of grief
3. Realization	Depression, apathy, fantasy	To adjust to life without the deceased
4. Acceptance	Readiness to engage in new activities and relationships	To relocate emotional energy elsewhere

of mourning that relate to each phase, encouraging the mourner and helper to recognize the potential for aiding the grief work in hand.

These four phases, with their associated features and tasks, can be summarized as shown in Table 2.1. Many factors will affect individual progress through these phases, which may take years to complete. Previous experience of loss and death, personality type, the relationship with the deceased, the nature of the death and support systems are all significant factors. For children, the attitudes and reactions of other family members, particularly parents, will largely determine their ability to cope with the loss.

The tasks of mourning

The tasks of mourning relate to the hard work involved in death, as in birth. Freud called bereavement 'grief work':

1. *Accepting the reality of the loss* is the first task and has to be done before the bereft feelings can be experienced. It is for this very reason that the psychological defence of denial comes into play, as protection against overwhelming trauma, and is initially useful. If the denial persists, however, by refusing to accept the facts or significance of the death, life without the deceased cannot be faced. Means of facing the loss include the viewing of the body and attendance at the funeral or other rituals. Seeing is believing at a gut level. Talking about the circumstances of the death, over and over again, is another important way of making it real.
2. *Experiencing the pain of grief* is the key task and, if not confronted, the pain will work itself out in another way, perhaps psychosomatically or through destructive behaviours. Most commonly, avoidance of grieving leads to depression. Grief may be expressed

publicly or privately, loudly or quietly, in words or gestures, but the important thing is giving expression to it somehow. The Irish wake and the use of keeners to lead Indian mourners are two examples of helping the bereaved to let go of their emotions. The 'stiff upper lip' British attitude serves only to maintain the natural resistance to pain. Being given permission to talk, weep and rage, and having a safe environment in which to do so, can be crucially important, for the professional carer as well as for the family. Feelings of anger or guilt can be very frightening, and acknowledgement that they exist helps to make them more manageable.

3. *Adjusting to life without the deceased* is a time of transition. Withdrawal from normal life seems necessary. It is experienced as a lonely time, usually accompanied by lethargy and regrets. The realization of how life will be without the loved one begins to sink in and many adjustments have to be faced. This is again a time for talking, also for reading and writing, to work through the meaning of what has happened, to try and make sense of the loss. Practical issues need to be resolved too, and new ways found of relating to the world.

4. *Relocating emotional energy elsewhere* signifies that the death and bereavement have been integrated into an ongoing life. It is an acceptance, however reluctant, that life is different, and a coming to terms with the futility of trying to retrieve the loss. The loved one is not forgotten, but has found a new place, which allows the bereaved to move on to new activities and relationships. There will be times of returning for a while to earlier phases, but generally the transition is complete. Those who do not complete the transition prefer to hold on to the lost attachment for fear there is nothing else.

Normal grief reactions

Normal grief reactions are defined by Worden as both clinically predictable and commonly experienced across the whole spectrum of the grieving process. A broad range of feelings, sensations, thoughts and behaviours fall within this description.

- Feelings of numbness, sadness, anger, guilt, anxiety, despair, loneliness, powerlessness, yearning, freedom, relief.
- Physical sensations of shock, fatigue, hollow stomach, aching limbs, dry mouth, breathlessness, tightness in the throat and chest, sensitivity to noise.
- Thoughts of disbelief, confusion, disorientation, obsessional preoccupation with the deceased, visual and auditory hallucinations.
- Behaviours such as sleep disturbance, lack of appetite, absentmindedness, crying, sighing, restless overactivity, searching, calling

out, lethargy, dreams, visiting the grave and special places, treasuring reminders and avoiding reminders.

It is important to note that although the intensity of these reactions can be alarming, both for the bereaved person and to those around, they can all be regarded as appropriate responses.

Complicated grief

Complicated grief is an umbrella term to describe reactions that deviate from the norm. Other terms used are chronic grief, abnormal grief and pathological grief. What is being indicated is a failure to grieve, which results in dysfunctional behaviour or illness. Progress towards healing the emotional wound of bereavement is blocked. Medical terms, which pepper the literature on complicated grieving such as 'morbidity', 'diagnosis' and 'symptoms', suggest a diseased state.

There are various classifications of complicated mourning.

- *Inhibited or delayed grief* denotes an inability to mourn and an avoidance of the painful feelings. For some reason the bereaved person is unable to accept the reality of the loss.
- *Distorted bereavement* describes an exaggerated aspect of grieving, commonly anger or guilt, which prevents the expression of other feelings such as sorrow and yearning. This is often linked to the sense of desertion when the relationship with the deceased was a very dependent one.
- *Chronic grief* is recognized in those who continue to grieve intensely and unremittingly long after the event. The bereaved person remains acutely distressed in a way that seems inappropriate and disabling. There is continued crying, anger, and idealization of the loved one.

In each of these patterns there is a denial of some aspects of the loss and a frustrated state of trying to hold on to the lost relationship.

Unhealthy outcomes of incomplete mourning

Denial, delay or suppression of some aspects of grief commonly lead to depression. Painful feelings that cannot be expressed are pushed down, and holding them down absorbs a lot of energy. The bereaved person presents with fatigue, loss of libido, irritability and other depressive symptoms. Suicidal impulses are usually associated with depression.

For some people, these painful feelings threaten to be so overwhelming that a high anxiety state is produced. Panic attacks and phobias may be associated reactions. Grief may be masked by various maladaptive or acting-out behaviours, which then become problematic in themselves. These include alcohol and other drug dependence, delinquent and criminal activity, inappropriate sexual behaviour and eating disorders.

Psychosomatic conditions may develop as a result of postbereavement stress that is not being expressed directly. This form of displaced pain often stimulates some aspect of the deceased person's illness or injury.

What causes complicated grieving?

The many factors involved can be grouped in four categories.

1. *Relationships.* Ambivalent relationships, such as the classic love/ hate relationship between some adolescents and parents, make for difficult grieving, particularly if the ambivalent feelings are not owned. The loss of such a relationship causes excessive amounts of either anger or guilt or both. Another kind of relationship that causes problems is the highly dependent one. This is often in the context of a child losing a parent at a crucial stage of dependence, but also relates to a parent losing a child who represented an extension of oneself. Sometimes the amount of 'unfinished business' between the deceased and the bereaved can inhibit mourning. In the case of an abusive relationship, the death will awaken any unspoken grievances, anger and guilt.

2. *Circumstances.* Certain circumstances in themselves preclude any satisfactory working out of grief. Obvious examples are the 'missing, presumed dead' loss in war, the lack of an identifiable body as the result of accident or murder and a situation involving multiple losses. Any uncertainty as to the cause of death leaves the bereaved uncertain how to react. When sudden death takes place in particularly horrific circumstances the resulting trauma may overwhelm the capacity to grieve.

3. *Personal factors.* These may relate to a history of difficult losses, which have an impact on current losses, or relate to a person's individual character. Early parenting, as well as early loss of a parent, are thought to be significant factors which affect later reactions to loss. Some personalities are vulnerable to difficulties because of an inability to cope with stress ('I can never cope'); and others because they are so self-sufficient as to be intolerant of any dependency and thus unable to acknowledge the significance of loss ('I can always cope'). This latter group includes people seen by society as 'strong' and in helping roles themselves, who find it hard to recognize and express their own needs.

4. *Social factors.* Grieving takes place in a social setting and an individual's reactions to loss will in some degree be dependent on the reactions of family, friends and the local community. Any socially unacceptable loss that carries some stigma, such as abortion, AIDS, abnormality and suicide, limits the amount of support available and increases the bereaved person's sense of isolation. The absence of a social support system is a key indicator of problematic grieving. Family and social support may be absent for other reasons, such as

moving into another geographical or cultural environment. There is an assumption that all those who live in Britain must conform to the practices established by Western civilization and the Christian tradition. This is particularly relevant to first generation immigrants from Eastern cultures, whose customs and rituals are not accommodated here. For the majority of Asian Indians, death is a family and community affair: the family construct the funeral bier on which the body is carried through the streets to the funeral pyre, which is lit by the family. During the first 12 days of mourning, the immediate family are expected to show their grief in public. Such traditions would hardly be tolerated in the West, where death is sanitized by coffins and crematorium curtains, and grief is a very private affair.

Grieving for a child

How adequate is the general bereavement theory when applied to the death of a child?

Attachment theory is obviously relevant to all forms of loss. It provides an understanding of the powerful and primitive forces at work when we grieve – the grief process. It also validates the intensity of the pain and protest reactions of bereaved parents. So much is invested in the child by the parent, and the mother/baby bonding is the primary attachment that forms the base of all significant relationships. In particular, the trauma, anxiety and depression caused by the loss of a baby before or at birth tend to be underestimated in our society. Appreciation of the strong attachments that can form even before birth should prevent this mother's experience, which is all too common:

'I had waited 12 years to have this baby. Then, in the last month things went wrong very quickly and I was in a nightmare. I knew she was dead before I went into labour. We called her Louise and she looked perfect, just as I'd imagined. I desperately wanted a girl, and I just knew she was going to be special. The consultant came round the day after she was born and said 'it' was just one of those things. He said that at least I had two teenage boys so it could have been worse, and I could go back to work after four weeks and resume intercourse after six. He seemed to have no idea what she meant to me'.

The features of grieving are also relevant to the loss of a child, as to any other bereavement. The same pattern of reactions is observable too in the anticipatory grief of parents of a terminally ill child. However, a model of stages and phases seems too rigid to describe the traumatic and chaotic disorganization that parents experience following the death of their child. Parents attending the Alder Centre have found comfort in sharing with others the *unpredictability* of their reactions. They report their puzzlement at how the full gamut of emotions return again and again. Typically the observation that 'only now has the reality sunk in' is repeated at intervals throughout the first year of bereavement, and possibly well into the second. The loss of one's child is a magnification of other losses. It is often so fundamental to one's sense of self, one's purpose and direction, that one's life has been turned upside down.

An alternative model

A pictorial approach to grief developed by Dr Richard Wilson, a consultant paediatrician at Kingston Hospital who has worked closely with bereaved parents, more accurately reflects the turmoil of reactions and unique experience of every individual. It depicts an unsuspecting oarsman rowing along the 'River of Life' who is suddenly plunged down the 'Waterfall of Bereavement' to the 'Whirlpool of Grief' below. The whirlpool carries one round and round, visiting the same emotions time and again, with the occasional respite in the shallows and the risk of being cast against the rocks. The time spent in this period of disorganization will vary, and some who have been washed up on a bank will choose to stay there. But when the time is right for reorganization, the 'River of Life' leads away from the whirlpool to calmer waters (Figure 2.1).

Figure 2.1: The Whirlpool of Grief

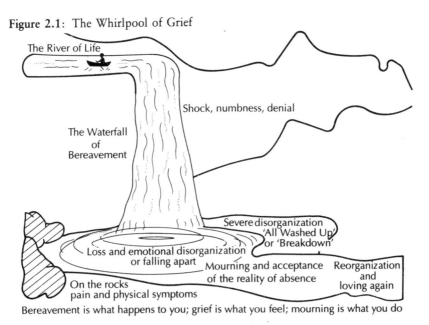

The River of Life

Shock, numbness, denial

The Waterfall of Bereavement

Severe disorganization 'All Washed Up' or 'Breakdown'

Loss and emotional disorganization or falling apart

Mourning and acceptance of the reality of absence

Reorganization and loving again

On the rocks pain and physical symptoms

Bereavement is what happens to you; grief is what you feel; mourning is what you do

Source: Richard Wilson, Kingston Hospital.

Those who have come across this analogy have found it helpful and an attractively simple model. These are Richard Wilson's comments about it:

> It may be a little fanciful. However, it is less rigid than suggesting that there are stages of grief which must be completed. People cannot be healed by shepherding them through a fixed treatment plan; however we may be of some assistance as they make their way along their own difficult and personal journey.
>
> Grief is a turbulent time, and although there may be precious periods of calm, violent emotions which had seemed to be over can return. They are innumerable and all valid. In grief there is a disorganization of life and thought and values, but most people are then able to reorganize their life in a new way. Although old emotions can always return in almost the same intensity, they do so less frequently and for shorter periods of time.

The value of this model is that it emphasizes the need to listen to parents rather than rely on a taught framework. Bereavement support requires skill and sensitivity rather than knowledge.

The concept of enduring grief

Resolution of grief is a difficult concept for parents: many would reject the idea that grieving for one's child can ever end, and some consciously choose to stay with the intensity of their early grief as a mark of loyalty to the child they can no longer care for. The saying 'time heals' holds a hollow promise for John, whose 10-year-old daughter Clare died during a heart operation, and who speaks here for a significant proportion of bereaved parents:

> 'When newcomers join us at the Centre, they remind us all of how we were not so long ago, and for me that's good. I don't ever want to leave that behind. I want to always be reminded of the intensity of what I felt, and time robs you of that.'

Bowlby and Parkes say that mourning is finished when a person completes the final phase of restitution, implying a restoration to a previous state. Worden prefers the more open-ended view that mourning is finished when the associated tasks are completed, and has no definitive timescale. Although rejecting attempts to set dates, he concludes (Worden, 1991: p. 18): 'In the loss of a close relationship I would be suspicious of any full resolution that takes under a year and, for many, two years is not too long.' He also quotes from Parkes's studies, which show that widows may take three to four years to re-establish stability in their lives. But he also warns us that the culmination of mourning will not be to a pregrief state and that reworking of grief may be required.

In fact, most of the research and literature is focused on spousal grief, which has to be amended when considering the loss of a child.

Peppers and Knapp coined the phrase 'shadow grief' to describe the burden of grief that mothers of children who died in infancy carry for the rest of their lives. The shadow may cast a black pall at special times, such as anniversaries, but is always in the background as an aching reminder of qualified joy. In ideal circumstances, this 'shadow grief' may resolve; but for most parents a sense of 'enduring sorrow' is both natural and normal.

So what is normal?

The outcome of bereavement is taken as the measure of what is normal and what is pathological. According to the standard bereavement theory, the grief experienced by most bereaved parents would be labelled as chronic, certainly, and probably as 'abnormal' in other respects.

A study of parents whose children had died on the Intensive Care Unit (ICU) at Great Ormond Street Hospital for Sick Children in London over a period of nine months measured the effects of their bereavement (Sumner et al., 1991). The study concluded that:

> Psychiatric disturbance was three times more likely in a group of parents who lost a child on an ICU than in a similar group whose child survived an ICU admission.

Identifying these parents as a high-risk group is important in terms of getting adequate resources for their support. However, the pathological label is unfortunate on two counts.

1. Parents who feel that their grief is abnormal may suffer in silence rather than risk a psychiatric label.
2. Those who provide support may have unrealistic expectations about the capacity of bereaved parents to return to a 'normal' functioning.

A revealing questionnaire conducted by the Alder Centre in 1991 showed that professionals and non-bereaved volunteers had a more optimistic view of outcome than either the bereaved parents they were supporting or parent volunteers. Again, the experience of the Alder Centre is that so-called pathological states of depression, anxiety and suicidal impulses are norms amongst bereaved parents. Surely the loss of a child falls into a category that is compared unfairly with other bereavements, especially when the loss is sudden and unexpected. Too often it is described as a subsection of bereavement situations, rather than being a state of bereavement with its own norms.

The quality of the parent–child bond is surely the most significant factor in regarding the nature of child bereavement. The parent–child relationship naturally contains many of the elements identified by Worden and others as indicators of complicated grief, in particular a high degree of dependence and ambivalence. Children also represent the gratification, or frustration, of basic psychological needs – for love, approval and acceptance.

Parents

The grieving of parents, then, is almost inevitably going to be complicated, and may never be resolved. In considering what the death of a child means to a parent, it has already been noted how many losses are involved. As well as the losses special to that unique relationship, parents have much to lose in terms of their own security in the world. As one parent put it 'When you lose your parents, you lose your past: when you lose a child, you lose your future.' The relationship between the parents will be tested, and the whole family system will be stressed.

Age of the child

The age of the child is a principal factor in the significance of the loss, although the death of a child at any age is untimely. A preterm or newborn baby has a fantasy existence for the parents and remains a dream-child in death. A baby who dies within the first year of life leaves the aching arms of a mother from whom he has hardly separated physically. At this age bonding with both parents (or principal carers) is likely to be at its most intense.

As the young child develops, so does its place in the family. Again, a first child will become central to the parents' emotional life. Sometimes a child takes on a special significance for one of the parents: a mother may feel that a particular child 'belongs' to her, or a father may identify strongly with one child as meeting his own needs. As the child becomes more of a real person, developing a separate identity, relationships become more complex. Ambivalent feelings and conflict inevitably affect the child-parent relationship in the teenage years. As one of the tasks of adolescence is to separate from parents and achieve independence, the death of a teenager is likely to leave in its wake a complicated web of unresolved feelings.

It is perhaps more straightforward for parents to adjust to the death of an adult child, when some degree of separation has taken place, although the grief will be just as intense. Older parents will be grieved that they did not die first.

Effects on parents

Effects on the individual parent will obviously vary according to the quality of the relationship with the child, personality, previous experience of loss and what kind of support is available. Parents are often affected by doubts of their sanity and their worth.

'Am I going mad?' is a usual response to the extreme distress and disorganization of the early months of mourning.
'Can I go on' is a usual response to the feelings of worthlessness and despair that make it hard to face another day.
'I'd like to join him' is a usual response to feelings that the child has deserted the parent, and the parent has failed the child.

The parenting role

Effects on the parenting role will obviously be dramatic when an only child dies. In the eyes of society, they are no longer parents, no longer a family. The direct line of genetic descent has come to an end. Where there are other children, parental grief is likely to be inhibited and tempered by their needs, which may cause resentment or relief. When the surviving children are young, or when other pregnancies quickly follow the bereavement, mothers in particular do not have the space and time to themselves to grieve and are vulnerable to depression. On the other hand, parents who find they can think only of the dead child have little interest or energy for their other children. They may be aware of this and feel guilty about it but it takes a huge effort to do otherwise. Women whose entire identity and self-esteem depend on motherhood may lose a vital sense of self, suffer chronic guilt and face a huge task of adjustment. Fathers who see themselves as the family providers and protectors will feel they have failed in their responsibility, and this may threaten their sense of manhood.

The marriage or partnership

Effects on the marriage or partnership will depend largely on the strength of the couple's relationship beforehand. Any needs that are not being met will be magnified by the loss and cause resentment, particularly if the child supplied some of those needs for one or other of the parents. Initially a reasonably open and trusting relationship will allow the parents to comfort each other, although as time goes on even the closest of couples find that grief separates them in some way – it is essentially a lonely experience. Two people cannot grieve at the same pace nor tend to each other's needs without sacrificing their own. One father put it this way: 'It's like both of you having flu at the same time. You feel so wretched that you can't help your partner.'

Another major factor is the different ways in which the partners may express their grief. Stereotypically the mother copes with her pain by crying and talking, while the father copes with his pain by being active and busy. These differences may be respected, but are more likely to cause resentment that the husband does not appear to be grieving or that the wife is draining him emotionally. They may turn to others for understanding and thus widen the rift. However it happens, a significant number of bereaved couples end up living separately, and most couples experience severe strains on their relationship. An Australian study by Nixon and Pearn (1977) found that marital breakdown occurred in 24% of families following the drowning of a child.

Dot, whose only child Christine died from cystic fibrosis, reflects here on how she and her husband grew apart after Christine's death:

> 'Bob and I started by grieving together, but after those first weeks in the depths of despair we couldn't keep in step. I'd look across at him and think, "He's not thinking about Christine at this moment, and so if I say something now, I will be invading his peace . . . let him have this break". But then as time went on, I realized that I could cope with my own very mixed emotions. In a way I was happier not to have to share them. I suppose in my own way I was shutting other people out, including Bob, but somehow that felt safer to me. I think that was the trigger point for grieving apart. Bob then threw himself into his work, and I was left to pick up the pieces of my life, and so our different ways of coping took us further apart. I think grief is such an individual thing that I don't believe you can grieve as a couple.'

John and Sue, whose second child David died of cancer, also found that they grieved in separate ways, but found a way of communicating their needs which strengthened their relationship. John explains:

> 'A major factor which helped to bind us together was our relationship with our daughter, Jane. Answering the questions of a three-year-old forced us to bring things out in the open for ourselves.'

Grandparents

The effects of losing a grandchild are often underestimated. The two-generation gap can free grandparents to indulge the child with the kind of attention and affection which creates a special bond between them. Grandchildren represent a continuing link with the future at a time of life when one is increasingly aware of one's own mortality. Grandparenting presents another opportunity to endow children with hopes and expectations, although often tempered by a more realistic view and more tolerant attitudes.

Some grandparents will have been involved directly with the care of the child, particularly when both parents are in employment outside the home or when a young mother is still living at home. In these cases the grandparent takes on a parenting role and the intensity of grief is more akin to that of the parent. Grandparents are also likely to be closely involved with the support of both child and parents in the case of terminal illness.

It is this dual role and relationship that causes most anguish to grandparents. They suffer their own grief, and are affected deeply by their own child's grief. They often feel helpless and inadequate in the support they can offer, frustrated by their inability to comfort and protect.

This was Diane's experience:

'Other people feel I shouldn't be grieving the way I am, because Anthony was only a grandson. We weren't just nanna and grandson, we were friends. In my case, I'm grieving not only for Anthony but for my daughter as well. I found I couldn't help her.'

She also writes movingly about the guilt which she felt:

'Guilty about what? Guilty that I am alive and my beautiful grandson, Anthony, is dead. Guilty because my daughter Julie, Anthony's mummy, is ill, torn apart by grief. Guilty because after Anthony died I sought help for myself. For the first time in my life, I put myself before anyone else. Why? Because I was in so much pain, I couldn't help anyone else.'

Siblings

Brothers and sisters have been called 'the forgotten mourners'. The effects of sibling loss on young children is not easily remembered or understood, and their needs are not always expressed directly. The age and developmental stage of the grieving child is an important factor, of course, but before looking at different age groups, what are the common factors affecting all siblings?

First, there is the parents' grief and the ways in which their reactions affect their other children. What happens at the time of the death and what the surviving children are told are both crucially important. At any age, a child will be affected by the parent's distress and made anxious by upheaval in the home and family. There is a natural inclination to protect children from witnessing their parents' grief. Yet it is essential for them to see their parents mourn, or they will believe that the dead child was not loved and fear that they would not be mourned either if they were to die.

Siblings are also affected by the impact on the family as a system and the balance of relationships within it. All are required to adjust to the void left by the dead child. One consequence may be that a surviving sibling 'takes the place' of the dead child, fulfilling a particular role with regard to one or both of the parents. Another possible outcome, in a situation where the dead child was intensely idealized by the parents, is that a sibling can become the scapegoat for parental anger and guilt. She finds herself competing with an angel, and is found wanting. Families that normally function by sharing feelings and being open about difficulties will fare better than those that avoid emotions. Families that already have disordered patterns and a history of conflict may be plunged into chaos by the traumatic loss of a child, with serious consequences for all family members.

At any age, siblings lose an ally, particularly when left as an only child. Sibling relationships tend to be ambivalent, with love and affection interwoven with resentment and rivalry. Whatever that balance, the sibling loses a playmate or companion, and someone to identify with in the generation struggle with the adult world. For twins and siblings of a similar age the natural bond is closer. Older siblings are likely to be left with feelings of responsibility and maybe irrational guilt that they could not protect their younger brother or sister. Younger siblings are left with a feeling of insecurity following the failure of their older brother or sister to pave the way to adulthood successfully.

Ages and stages

The age of the sibling is seen as a key factor in anticipating the child's experience of grief, and so provides guidance as to what to say and do. Often, the adults involved will be wary of exposing a young child to information or experiences to which she is assumed to be 'too young to understand'. Before going on to describe the features relevant to age groups, it is important to note that children do not automatically reach a new level of understanding on a birthday! Children mature at different rates, and any significant loss may cause regression to a previous stage of development: for example, an eight-year-old will cling to mother again like a four-year-old.

It is also helpful to remember that knowledge comes through experience: what a child understands depends more on her previous experience of the world than on her age.

A word of caution about how adults perceive children, because the way we communicate our understanding is determined by the level of language we use. Children are exposed to images of death, via the media and religious symbolism, long before they have the words to describe them. Therefore the tendency is always to underestimate what a child can understand. At the same time, a child's emotional immaturity restricts the ability to cope with intense distress for long periods. This leads to the tendency to underestimate the effects of the bereavement.

Nought to two

The beginnings of grief and mourning can be seen as young as six months, when the baby certainly responds to the disappearance of close attachment figures. These are not likely to include a sibling, unless a twin or older parental figure. An 18-month-old baby who watches a caterpillar lying still after being squashed and says 'no more', is demonstrating a rudimentary understanding of death.

Two to five years

During this time a child develops the power of fantasy to deal with an increasingly difficult world. Magical thinking can make dangerous things safer, so games like cowboys and indians, 'bang bang, you're dead', are played out projections. If a sibling dies, there is a real danger that the child will believe that her destructive fantasies have come true. Even the most loving of children resents the intrusion of a younger sibling and will have wished him away. Such fears are likely to be kept hidden, so reassurance that the child is in no way to blame for the death needs to be offered. Similarly, the child may fear that her own death is imminent, particularly if the death was sudden and difficult to explain.

Sugar-pill explanations need to be avoided when it comes to answering questions about death and what happens after death. As children of this age think in literal, concrete terms, euphemisms such as 'gone to heaven' or 'gone to sleep' can cause confusion and distress.

Children in this age range are often actively excluded from the knowledge of a sibling's fatal illness, in the mistaken belief this will protect them from pain. Rather, the child's fantasies will build on the mystery, which becomes more frightening than the truth. The same applies to exclusion from hospital visits and funeral rites: the child will make up what she does not see, so that careful consideration needs to be given as to what information to offer and how to give it.

In fact, children of this age tend to take things very much in their stride in a way that can seem hurtful to parents. On being told about the stillbirth of a baby brother, one five-year-old girl's response was to ask for the baby clothes for her doll. Very practical! It is tempting to project adult feelings onto children. Any powerful feelings belonging to a child of this age are not sustained and show in short bursts.

Five to eight

By the age of eight most children develop an understanding of death as having a cause, of being irreversible and as something that can happen to anyone, even the child herself. The child is able to convey more of her understanding verbally, although denial of feelings is a natural defence and outwardly the child may seem unaffected. The development of conscience heightens the sense of guilt, and irrational links are often made between 'naughty' behaviour towards a younger sibling who then dies.

Eight to 12

The child's understanding of the finality of death is now nearly equivalent to that of an adult, although abstract concepts may still be difficult.

The most important factor is the growing realization of the possibility of the child's own death and the fear this engenders. Grief and mourning for a lost sibling may therefore be inhibited. When extreme guilt and fear is shown in depressive withdrawal or disturbed reactions to illness, including the development of symptoms belonging to the dead sibling's condition, specialist help is indicated to confront any distorted or confused thoughts.

Adolescence

This period of turbulence is marked by anxieties about the future and reluctance to face the reality of death. Relationships with siblings are now more complex, with mixed feelings of envy and pride. The adolescent who loved and valued her sibling will be deeply affected, but her own grief is often deferred to that of the parents or the family as a whole. This may stem from a desire to protect her parents, although in even the closest of families teenagers more naturally turn to friends to talk about feelings.

A group of teenagers who met at the Alder Centre shared common feelings of depression, confusion and lack of confidence. They identified problems with sleep and concentration, and reported a lack of understanding from schoolteachers and schoolmates. Mike, whose younger brother Philip died after a heart operation, explained his motivation in coming to the group:

'I needed somewhere to go where I could fully express what I was feeling in front of people I could relate to, something which was hard to do in front of my parents or my friends.'

Most common anxieties of grieving siblings

Across the board, the most common anxieties of siblings can be summarized crudely as:

'Did I cause it?'
'Will I die too?'
'Who now cares for me?'

Key needs of siblings are for information, reassurance, understanding and attention.

It is important to remember that the complex effects of the *secondary bereavements* experienced by the child, such as the loss of security and diminished attention from parents, can be more traumatic than the loss of the sibling.

Carers

This term includes the wide variety of people involved in the care of the terminally ill child and the bereaved family. Carers will themselves be affected by the child's death. The involvement may be in a professional or voluntary capacity, and may be part and parcel of the work role or incidental to it.

For the professional carer, there is an overwhelming sense of helplessness when, in spite of all one's training and dedicated care, a child's life is lost. However, for those who work closely with the family, there is a lot of job fulfilment in knowing how their support is valued. The stresses and satisfactions associated with various roles are considered in Chapter 3.

It can be difficult to allow for personal feelings within a professional role, which requires a certain detachment. When the child concerned has anything in common with one of the carer's own children – for instance the same name, age or school – then the carer will make this connection, either consciously or unconsciously.

The ways in which carers are affected are perhaps best illustrated by giving an example from those who first become involved: (1) before the death; (2) at the time of the death; and (3) after the death.

1. Jenny is a sister attached to the cystic fibrosis ward of a children's hospital. All the children in her care will die, probably in late adolescence or early adulthood. Jenny has known these children from diagnosis in infancy, and is affected at that time by the shock and anger that mark the beginning of the parents' grief. Over the years she becomes part of the extended family, sharing their hopes and fears, advising and supporting the parents in their care of the child. The child becomes more of a friend than a patient, and may share thoughts and feelings with Jenny that cannot be risked with parents. During the final illness, Jenny seeks to keep the child comfortable and helps the family prepare for the death. The death of the child is a personal loss for Jenny, too, and she must handle her grief alongside her responsibilities to other staff and other patients. The empathy and compassion required for this work forbid a distancing approach and are emotionally draining. Support and renewal are essential.

2. Ron is a paramedic in the ambulance service. As he is often the first professional to arrive on the scene, he is regarded as a saviour and source of hope. It feels like a failure to confirm death instead. His way of coping with emergency is to take action, so it goes against the grain to stay and talk to parents after a cot death. Ron's professionalism carries him through at the time and immediately afterwards – his next call may be a maternity call – so it is later when the reactions set in. He feels useless, physically shaky and churned up inside. He is deeply affected by the thought that one of his three children could die, and is aware of being more affectionate and protective towards them as a result.

3. Sarah is a health visitor with three bereaved families on her caseload, as well as several mothers suffering depression following miscarriage. She uses her counselling skills to show empathy with the bereaved, but it is stressful trying to say the right things and she has no supervision or support to deal with her feelings of helplessness. This means that she takes her feelings home with her, but finds it difficult to share them. She doesn't think her family want to hear about babies dying. However, she has a good friend who lost a baby herself, and she reassures Sarah about the real support she is giving just by visiting the families. Sarah is also talking to a colleague in another district about setting up a supervision group.

Rituals

Some features particular to the death of a child affect the bereavement and mourning rituals. These may be practical differences related to the age of the child, cultural differences related to the status of the child or differences of emphasis to do with the special relationship between parent and child.

Given the enduring nature of parental grief, strongly marked by feelings of failure and guilt, it is very important to parents that they 'do their best' for their child after death, which is one aspect of bereavement rituals. For themselves, and for others too, rituals also help to make the loss real and aid the mourning tasks. A third function of rituals is to provide social recognition of the death and public expression of the emotions aroused.

At the time of the death

Most religious faiths have rites that are performed with the aid of a priest, minister or holy person, to prepare the dying for the life to come and to lay the dead to rest.

Common to those of all faiths, and those with none, is the need to say goodbye to the child, which is in itself a ritual. Seeing, touching, holding and talking to the child all have added significance when the death was unexpected and sudden, and when perinatal death involves saying hello as well as goodbye.

Not all believers in a particular religion keep the same observance of traditional rituals, although it is important to be aware of orthodox practice. For example, distress may be caused to both the Muslim and Hindu family if a child's body is touched after death by a non-believer, although disposable gloves may be used if the family are unable to prepare the body themselves. Removing a lock of hair would be offensive to Muslims, and strict adherents of Islam may discipline themselves to show no emotion at the death of their child, believing it to be the will of Allah. For an Orthodox Jewish child, the first acts of shutting the eyes, binding up the jaw and laying the arms straight are traditionally done by a family member.

The legal ritual of registering the death, and the practical task of informing friends, family and officialdom that the child has died, are ways in which the reality of bereavement is faced and rehearsed. The absence of formal rituals such as registration is much regretted by those whose baby died before the legal age of viability.

Funeral rites

The placing of mementoes such as a favourite toy in the coffin or on the grave is a powerful symbol of the continuing link between parent and child beyond the grave. Participation in the funeral rites is important to all those who are significantly affected by the death. The question of whether young children should attend the funeral is for the parents to decide and will be considered in more detail in Chapter 5. Those who do not attend can participate in other ways, for example by being involved in decision-making about the form of service, choice of music and so on.

In normal circumstances, Jewish and Muslim funerals take place within 24 hours of the death, and Hindus prefer the funeral to take place as soon as possible. If delay is unavoidable, the reasons need to be carefully explained. Coroners' officers will make special arrangements if a post-mortem is required, so that the funeral is not unduly delayed.

After the funeral

Of all the major religions, Islam upholds the most exacting mourning rituals. The family stays at home for the first three days, and food is brought in by relatives. Strict mourning lasts for 40 days, after which the grave is visited on Fridays. Traditional Hindu mourning is a communal affair, with constant visiting of extended family and neighbours. During the first 12 days after the funeral, ritualistic mourning takes place in the family home, led by an experienced female relative, to encourage the open expression of grief.

Having a place to visit, whether it be a grave or garden of remembrance, provides a continuing ritual for the expression of grief. The intense yearning to be physically close to the child again can be so great as to engender fantasies of digging up the coffin. Initially life may only be bearable if sustained by daily visits to the grave to reassure the child of continuing love and care. Later, the placing of the headstone is another formal ritual to mark the permanence of death.

Keeping the child's name alive is a primary concern for parents, and at least a temporary concern for others too.

Memorial ceremonies provide an opportunity for the child's school to celebrate the child's life and mourn his loss. Family, school and the local community may choose a form of commemoration, such as an award or dedication, or may embark on fund-raising activities to benefit an organization or area of research associated with the child.

Photographs and other mementoes may be avoided initially but eventually treasured. Sorting through the child's possessions is a painful business and may be long delayed. The distribution of mementoes in the form of toys and clothes amongst family and friends is usually much appreciated, as these are transitional objects linking the past to the future. Sadly, in the case of sudden death, there may be a superstitious reluctance for friends to accept anything belonging to the child.

Clearing the child's room is another important milestone and not one to be hurried. The choice of when it feels right to do this is an individual one and should be left entirely to the parents.

Anniversaries of birth and death and special times all present opportunities to take stock of the journey through grief and to remember the child in a special way. Inscriptions in a Book of Remembrance are particularly valued by those who have few tangible reminders. Similarly, a joint memorial service, such as the annual Candle Service at Liverpool, when a candle is lit for every named child, is another way of using ritual to celebrate life as well as to mourn death.

References

Bowlby J (1991) *Attachment and loss*, vol 1, 2nd edn. Penguin, Harmondsworth.

Nixon J and Pearn J (1977) Emotional sequelae of parents and sibs following the drowning of a child. *Australian & New Zealand Journal of Psychiatry*, **11**, 265–8.

Parkes CM (1972) *Bereavement*. Tavistock Press, London.

Peppers LG and Knapp RJ (1980) *Motherhood and mourning*. Praeger, New York.

Sumner M *et al.* (1991) Loss on a paediatric intensive care unit: parental reactions. *Care of the Critically Ill*, 7(2), 64–6.

Worden JW (1991) *Grief counselling and grief therapy*, 2nd edn. Tavistock/Routledge, London.

Further reading

Green J (1991) Death with dignity: meeting the spiritual needs of patients in a multi-cultural society. *Nursing Times*.

Neuberger J (1987) *Caring for dying people of different faiths*. Austen Cornish, London.

SECTION 2
Good Practice Guidelines

3 Professional roles

Attention is now focused on the roles and functions of various groups according to job title. Some, like the paediatric intensive care nurse or funeral director, have an essential role to play and will encounter the death of a child as part and parcel of their work. Others, such as the registrar of births, marriages and deaths, will have a single and functional contact with many bereaved families, while health visitors and social workers are likely to be involved in ongoing support. GPs and clergy may fill a key supportive role, although only rarely over a lifetime career. Ambulance and police personnel are in the front line in emergency situations, and their initial reactions can do much to help or hinder parents. Teachers seldom deal with the death of a child, and when they do it is in a peripheral way, but they too can perform significant functions and be profoundly affected.

Whatever the level of involvement, it is hoped that this chapter will give information, reassurance and confidence. Points of likely involvement with the terminally ill child or bereaved family will be identified and linked to the possible tasks to be undertaken. Examples of good practice will be illustrated by drawing on the experience of families and individual professionals.

Different professions are considered alphabetically. If this chapter is being used for reference, the reader's attention is drawn to the general principles, which apply to everyone, in Chapter 4.

Ambulance personnel

Involvement

Ambulance personnel are often the first emergency responders on the scene, minutes after the fatal accident, onset of acute illness or discovery of the dead child. The way they carry out their duties can make a significant contribution to how the family copes subsequently. Ambulance crews are trained in resuscitation and, by 1994, every crew should include a paramedic, who is qualified to administer drugs. One ambulance technician in London had dealt with 10 child deaths in five years: another could recall four in 18 years. The typical pattern of response is a 999 call through the radio control system, administering resuscitation or treatment at the scene as appropriate and transporting the child to the hospital accident and emergency department, or directly to the mortuary if the death has been certified at home.

Function

The arrival of the ambulance is seen as a source of hope, and the ambulance officer as a saviour. When there is indeed hope of the child's life being saved, the obvious priority is emergency treatment and hospitalization. When the child is already dead, however, it is usually the ambulance officer who is the first professional to confirm the fact. It is necessary for the parents to hear this unambiguous statement if they are to begin to take in the reality of what has happened. The priority is now the care and comfort of the parents and family.

In the case of sudden death at home, the ambulance crew will have a vital role to play in co-ordinating initial support. This may involve contacting the other parent, relatives, GP, clergy and explaining why the police must attend. As the first on the scene after a cot death, their reassurance to parents that the death was not preventable is invaluable.

Concerns

As ambulance personnel are trained for action, it is hard to deal with the feelings of uselessness when the child has died at home. They are faced with extreme family reactions, which are unpredictable. Later, they have their own reactions to deal with, including 'there but for the grace of God goes one of mine'. If they seek help to come to terms with their own feelings over and above the informal support available from colleagues, they risk being seen as weak and inadequate. Perhaps the greatest fear is being called to a home death that involves suspected child abuse. This situation calls for great restraint to cope with the anger that arises when the basic instinct of saving life has been betrayed.

Good practice

The following pointers have been drawn from the experience of a county training officer in the ambulance service and a reference manual published by the Irish Sudden Infant Death Association:

> Sensitivity, common sense and good communication skills are valuable for the initial support of parents immediately after the death. These are shown by:
> - treating the child with respect and referring to him by name
> - offering practical help and comfort to the family
> - being generous with time and not hurrying a dead child away
> - explaining the bodily changes which may occur during or after the dying process, such as discoloration

- explaining what will happen and where, reassuring parents that they can see and hold the child again at hospital
- always taking mother or nearest relative with the child in the ambulance and encouraging her to hold the child.

Support for personnel affected by distress and trauma is part of building up good working practices and relationships with fellow officers and other colleagues in the health service.

Clergy

Involvement

Many families that give little or no active support to their church will fall back on the traditional beliefs and rituals of their culture. Thus the leader of the local religious community, whether priest, minister, imam or rabbi, is nearly always involved at the time of the death or soon after. Hospital chaplains are often involved before the death of a terminally ill child, building up supportive relationships with both families and staff. In many hospitals the chaplain is on call to attend to parents of a child who has been brought into casualty or intensive care, as part of a co-ordinated team response. In maternity hospitals, the chaplain is closely involved, and will usually conduct the funeral.

Most clergy offer their pastoral support by visiting the family as soon as they hear of the death of a child in their area, often from the undertaker, and continue to visit for as long as the family wish. The priest or minister who has an accumulated knowledge of the family history is ideally placed to receive the expression of grief.

However, now that fewer than one in four babies is baptized into the Church of England, the reality is that the spiritual meaning of the church is no longer relevant to the majority.

Function

The hospital chaplain is an important source of emotional support for many parents, some of whom will derive comfort from having their young infant baptized or receiving a blessing.

Unless the family already has an allegiance to a particular church, the parochial role is restricted to conducting the funeral service. John, an Anglican priest in a town parish, describes himself as a 'necessary functionary' for death rituals in a secular society. He makes a point of visiting the family as soon as possible, 'just to listen and act as a buffer for the injustice and anger they feel'. He has learned that there is nothing he can say in answer to the question 'Why has God done this to my innocent child?' except to acknowledge the distress. Later, perhaps, is the time for engaging with the family in a spiritual search for meaning, but for now he resists the platitudes of false comfort. Practically speaking, he can advise the family of their options and funeral arrangements, and help them to make informed choices. Parish clergy are in a good position to slow down well-meaning relatives who rush parents into hasty decisions.

Concerns

As the traditional role of the church becomes eroded, there are increasing dilemmas posed by the trend towards essentially humanist funerals. Family requests for the inclusion of popular music and secular readings may be seen as undermining the religious siginificance of the funeral service. Clergy are as subject to stress as anyone in the face of tragedy and may feel more exposed than most to the extent of human suffering. 'I try not to get over-involved', one priest told me, 'but the pathos of some cases just gets to me. . .'. Not all clergy are supported by an understanding spouse or fellow priest.

Confidentiality is an important issue, particularly for hospital chaplains, and may add to the stresses.

Good practice

David and Glenda were plunged into a nightmare when their three-year-old daughter, Stacey, suffered unsuspected heart problems during a minor nose operation and died after some hours in intensive care. The Catholic chaplain who was called to give a last blessing to Stacey stayed to comfort the shocked and angry parents and later took them home in his car. Glenda recalls:

> 'He was really good with Dave, who kept on at him about God letting Stacey die. He seemed to understand, and said we had every right to be angry.'

Clergy who are experienced in this area of grief say that expressions of sympathy need to be carefully chosen. Talking of 'God's will' or 'an angel in heaven' is not helpful. Parents of babies who have not been baptized need reassurance that Christian theology no longer sees this as an exclusion from God's grace. Similarly, parents who blame themselves need reassurance that their child's death is not a punishment.

Funeral directors

Involvement

Although legally there is nothing to stop parents managing the child's funeral themselves, nearly all will engage a funeral director to do this.

Contact is usually made within hours of the death. Those firms which offer a free basic service in the event of a child's death tend to take a special pride in this very sensitive part of their work.

Function

In the first interview with the parents, the funeral director or receptionist gives information about options and requires answers to difficult questions. Is a burial or cremation preferred? When is the funeral to be? Where will the child's body lie meanwhile? While always respecting the parents' wishes, the undertaker may offer points of view the parents had not considered: in determining burial or cremation, what happens if they move house in a few years? Many parents do not know what they can and cannot do, and may need encouragement to help to dress the child, to take the child out of the coffin or to have the child at home for a while.

In preparing the body for the coffin, special care is taken to present the baby or child in the most natural and attractive way. Photos, handprints and a piece of hair are usually offered to parents.

Male relatives often wish to carry the coffin themselves, which seems more appropriate when the child is young and the coffin small. If preferred, the funeral director and staff will take responsibility for this and other practical tasks, thus freeing the family to give way to their grief.

Concerns

Keeping the balance between compassion and professional detachment can be difficult. Nothing affects staff so much as the preparation of a young child for the coffin, and they will take enormous trouble to do their best for the family. The first interview with shocked and distraught parents can be very stressful.

Good practice

A funeral director with many years' experience believes the guiding principle should be to involve the family in the funeral preparations as much as possible:

'I always try to take my instructions from the parents themselves, and encourage them to see and hold the child as often as they wish. If parents are reluctant to take their baby out of the coffin, I hold the baby myself first, to give them confidence and to show my respect.'

Parents should not be rushed into making hasty decisions about funeral arrangements, and value advice about different options, ranging from a full church service to a simple ceremony in the home. The option of opening a new family grave is an important consideration for parents who eventually wish to be laid to rest in the same place as their child.

General practitioners

Involvement

Typically a doctor in general practice will deal with a child death every few years, usually in traumatic circumstances. An urban practice of three GPs at Haslington in Cheshire, serving a population of 7500, recorded seven deaths of under 21s over a period of seven years (Table 3.1). There is obviously a greater prevalence of loss by miscarriage, termination and perinatal deaths.

Table 3.1 Seven deaths in an urban practice (1985–1991)

Sex	Age	Cause	Year
M	19	Suicide	1985
M	1	Road accident	1985
F	13	Road accident	1986
M	16	Status asthmaticus	1988
F	14	Road accident	1988
F	20	Cystic fibrosis	1989
F	17	Road accident	1991

Function

The GP is a primary care manager, a central reference point of all community health care, and, as such, has a co-ordinating role. Assessment, treatment and referral are key functions. The GP will be a point of first contact for women who miscarry or seek termination of pregnancy. The GP's help is often sought in going through medical reports following a perinatal death. At the time of bereavement, the GP may be called on to alleviate post-trauma distress, and parents certainly appreciate a home visit at this time, particularly following a cot death. The GP provides medical information and advice. In the early days a mild sedative may be prescribed to help with sleep disturbance. Later, treatment of chronic stress and depression will range from advice to psychiatric referral, but in most cases will include some counselling and/or drugs, depending on the GP's resources and approach to mental health. Measures of healthy grieving are the frequency of visits to the practice centre, the nature of presenting symptoms, and the ability to return to work. As GPs are required to confirm fitness to work, they are in an excellent position to monitor the situation. They also provide continuity for the family and are readily accessible when other supports have fallen away. Record-keeping is an important function for providing this continuity of care, enabling the GP to relate behaviour or symptoms to previous losses.

Concerns

Lack of formal preparation and infrequent incidence of child death mean that the GP will have to call on inner resources. Traditional attitudes in the medical profession make it hard to deal with feelings of helplessness and inadequacy when a child dies. It goes against the grain for some doctors to be as open as parents would like, and many are more comfortable with sharing clinical detail than giving emotional support. Similarly, the traditional independence of doctors makes it hard to seek professional support and advice for themselves. Medical training and hospital work encourage the attitude that a doctor can cope with anything: in general practice a doctor is indeed expected to cope with everything, frequently switching from mundane to emotionally demanding tasks. On a practical level, GPs who are motivated to offer direct support have to guard their time and commitment priorities, both in the surgery and in terms of home visiting.

GPs may be subject to irrational criticism from parents. For example, it is a general pattern that parents change to another doctor after a cot death.

Good practice

In responding to a sudden death for the first time, the GP may welcome the following pointers as being valued by families.

- Showing that you care and sharing your feelings is much appreciated by parents.
- When presented with a dead child clearly beyond resuscitation, remember the value of parents being with their child *for as long as they wish* before handing over to the coroner.
- Families will welcome your reassurance that grieving is a gradual process that cannot be hurried, and that you and your team are available for ongoing support.
- In prescribing drugs to alleviate distress, be aware that many parents later regret taking antidepressants or other drugs that impede decision making and delay grieving, and prefer something to induce sleep.
- Advise parents of likely reactions, both physical and emotional, and reassure them of the normality of such symptoms as aching arms, distressing dreams, hearing the child's voice, loss of appetite and libido, anger and guilt.

- Encourage siblings to be involved by informing parents of the possible benefits of brothers and sisters seeing the dead child and attending the funeral.
- Explain practicalities, like the coroner's role, registering the death, funeral options.

Finally, these are the comments of a senior partner in a busy inner-city general practice:

'We all set ouselves high standards, so we may see a child's death as a personal failure. It is important to acknowledge and deal with these feelings. Our professional defences shouldn't get in the way of letting parents see our anxiety, uncertainty or sadness. Also, as a male GP, I can gently challenge the stereotypical father's need to 'be strong'. Overall, the most important thing is to be there for the family, not necessarily to do something. *Parents require human contact more than cold professionalism.'*

Health visitors

Involvement

Where long-term illness or disability leads to death, the health visitor will already be involved with the family, perhaps liaising with other agencies to provide nursery places for siblings, with benefit officers and with support organizations. She has a pivotal role in the communication protocol that follows childhood death. More districts and trusts are now publishing written procedures to formalize existing systems in which the health visitor is responsible for disseminating information from the hospital to the school, community health services and hospital staff. The health visitor has access to medical records and information about the family, knowledge of the community and local resources.

Involvement is immediate as well as automatic, and contact is made with the family as soon as the health visitor is informed of the death, possibly the same day. If the family is known, it may be appropriate to attend the funeral. Follow-up visits may continue up to the first anniversary, depending on the wishes of the parents.

Function

Immediate support on a practical level may include co-ordinating services, explaining procedures, liaising with the GP and providing medical information. Although health visitors are trained to give advice and help, in this situation they are also required to be active listeners, allowing the family to talk through their feelings. Their unique position in the community can provide excellent opportunities for addressing the needs of siblings, grandparents and the concerns of other families following a sudden death.

Follow-up after hospital visits is offered to parents, to go over the medical issues. Advice may be sought about surviving siblings and subsequent children. Mothers who are isolated may need a lot of emotional support, facing the health visitor with the dilemma of whether preventive mental health work is consistent with the role and caseload. The level of continuing support will depend partly on the individual's confidence in counselling skills and access to supervision. Referrals to other agencies for further help may be considered appropriate.

Concerns

In areas where there is no established protocol for health visitor liaison, there is always the anxiety about a loophole in communication. The resulting distress to parents when, say, a routine appointment arrives for the dead child, is deeply embarrassing. In the case of sudden death from SIDS or acute illness, the health visitor may be left with doubts and self blame: was there some sign or symptom that was missed, and were visits frequent enough?

Apprehension at the emotional turmoil of the bereaved family and how one will be affected personally is stressful. In visiting the home alone, the health visitor can take on some of the family's feelings of isolation and may well bear the brunt of parental feelings of guilt and blame, and be faced with very difficult questions with no easy answers.

There may be no support structure or formal supervision to help deal with personal reactions and assess appropriate levels of involvement. Where a need for further help for the family is identified, there may be a lack of local counselling and befriending resources.

Good practice

Detailed guidelines are to be found in leaflets published by the Foundation for the Study of Infant Death and the Scottish Cot Death Trust. The following advice is taken from discussions with several experienced professionals from different areas.

- Be sensitive to the parents' needs and go at their pace, being supportive without taking over.
- Avoid saying anything that implies judgement or criticism of the child's care.
- Be prepared to listen; share feelings and memories.
- Be there for *all* the family, including siblings and grandparents.

- Do not give up visiting for fear of intruding (unless requested to do so): continue telephone contact and remember anniversaries.
- Familiarize yourself with procedures in your area regarding hospitals, police, funeral arrangements, social services; and research local and national bereavement resources.

A health visitor provides this recent example of how her clinic supported the young mother of a four-month-old cot death baby:

'As a single parent with three other young children, Gwen needed a lot of support. My colleague was frustrated that Gwen was unwilling to do all the things advised for healthy grieving, like visiting the baby in the hospital, dressing him, having a photograph and so on. We talked it through as a team, and suggested to my colleague that there might be other members of the family who could be involved, and in fact two of Gwen's sisters were keen to help dress the baby and sort out the funeral and that's what happened. It was important for the family to be in charge.'

Hospital doctors

Involvement

Doctors may be involved in the casualty department, both at children's hospitals and at general hospitals, where they see the victims of accidents, of self-inflicted injuries and of emergency situations. Another obvious area is the intensive care unit, where, by definition, the illness is critical. Deaths occur more rarely on other hospital wards, such as from terminal pneumonia in a child with a chronic disability, or as the outcome of malignant disease and other life-threatening conditions. Here the consultant will already be a familiar and important person to the child and family, and may have been involved from the time of diagnosis, when grieving begins for many parents. Bereavement issues are also relevant to doctors involved with neonates, stillbirths and terminations for fetal abnormalities.

Function

As well as being responsible for the medical treatment of disease, doctors are concerned with the overall care of the patient, and for paediatricians the patient equals child *and* family. In the case of terminal illness, the consultant has the task of communicating the diagnosis, of explaining the progression of the condition, and keeping parents informed so that joint decisions can be made about treatment choices. This may include the crucial choice between active treatment and palliative care.

The doctor confirms the death, and if the parents are not present at the time, is likely to be the one to inform them. If the death is sudden, another task is to explain the legal process and possibility of a post-mortem. Explanations are required regarding the circumstances that have caused the death, and at this time parents need to know that they will have the opportunity of subsequent meetings to discuss post-mortem reports, answer questions relating to siblings, future children, genetic implications and future support resources. Some doctors offer routine home or hospital visits for such meetings.

At the time of death, the doctor needs to ensure that immediate support for the family is available from the social services department, chaplain or other designated staff. In the case of the death of a young infant, other practicalities include the control of pain and lactation and help with sleep.

In all deaths, there is a communication role, to liaise with the GP, health visitor and, in certain circumstances, with the community medicine specialist.

Concerns

Newly qualified doctors may find it hard to deal with young parents and older children because of their similarity in age.

Medical ethics are involved in some issues, such as:

- whether and when resuscitation efforts should cease
- whether active treatment should give way to palliative care
- when life-support systems should be withdrawn
- the use of donor organs.

Resources can become an overriding concern. Consultants who wish to improve facilities for the child's family, or introduce policies that allow greater parental involvement, will find themselves arguing against colleagues who see death as a non-medical issue.

Professionalism and personal feelings may be in conflict, causing anxiety about one's ability to handle the situation appropriately. Should feelings be shown, uncertainties admitted? How does one develop the skills and sensitivity needed to talk to bereaved parents? And where does the healer go for healing and support?

Good practice

Parents commonly identify several points relating specifically to hospital doctors.

- Even if the consultant was not present at the death, parents appreciated the consultant visiting them to acknowledge the death.

- Knowing and using the child's name, and looking the parents straight in the eye, conveyed respect.
- Expressing regret and appropriate use of touch conveyed real caring.

John Sills, a consultant paediatrician at Alder Hey Hospital, Liverpool, offers this advice to junior doctors working in casualty or intensive care:

'Basically they should show that they care about what has happened, that they respect the child and the family, and that they are there to answer questions. If the death is relatively non-acute they should keep the parents informed, and should liaise with their senior colleagues about what is happening.'

Richard Wilson, consultant paediatrician at Kingston Hospital, is widely respected for his work with bereaved families. These are his comments:

'We cannot make the situation better, but we may make it worse, and we must learn to avoid doing so. But we do care and are moved by events. As professionals we want to help, yet difficulties arise in distinguishing between our emotions and needs and those of the parents. We must acknowledge our personal feelings but not let them overwhelm our professional role. The family has need of our help, but we give it not as experts but almost as passers-by whom they have allowed in. There must be organization and guidelines, but we should have some understanding of ourselves, for only then can we be of use.

When we meet bereaved parents it is important to recognize the individuality of each situation, to know a little theory, to have tips – which come essentially from parents – on what can and cannot be done, to decide our own role, and in particular develop our ability to listen.'

Nurses

Involvement

All the areas quoted above for hospital doctors will also apply to hospital nurses. The primary nurse, a named nurse on the ward with whom parents can identify, will have a very close involvement with child and family. In the case of death after chronic illness, nurses are likely to have built up intimate relationships over many years. Neonatal nurses naturally become very attached to the babies in their care.

As a member of a primary health care team in the community, the nurse will be known to the family of a child who is terminally ill with cancer or a congenital abnormality.

Function

The nurse in casualty will form part of the emergency care team and, when the child dies, will have specific tasks relating to the laying out of the body. A senior nurse takes on responsibility for looking after the parents. Intensive care nurses are similarly required to carry out different roles, of technician before the death and comforter afterwards. Palliative care nurses work to ensure the control of pain and to see the child is comfortable.

Overall, the nurse administers and monitors the care plan and has a pivotal role regarding communication between parents and consultants. Whether the child dies at home or hospital, the parents are always seen as the main carers, and the professional role is advising and supporting them. Hospital nurses tend to become experts in disease, while community nurses develop expertise in ongoing support.

Concerns

The need for staff support is a big issue. Road traffic accidents and cot deaths are particularly harrowing, especially when the child is unmarked and looks perfectly normal. The laying out should not be done alone. Being with bereaved parents in the rawness of their grief is very stressful and emotionally draining. In some hospitals now there is a trained staff counsellor as well as peer support.

Management issues such as staffing quotas and time allocation create extra pressures. A ward nurse cannot give two hours to be with newly bereaved parents unless this is a priority for management too.

Many nurses are concerned with what to say to a dying child and how to answer their questions, especially when parents seek to protect them from the truth. Close contact can draw the professional into family friction and squabbles.

Community paediatric nurses can feel quite isolated if there is no built-in support, particularly if a home death happens at a weekend when hospital support systems are limited.

Good practice

Discussions with nurses experienced in accident and emergency, intensive care and palliative care highlight the importance of training in interpersonal skills to deal with the emotional demands of working with loss and grief. General guidelines which emerge are:

- be yourself: this includes being prepared to show feelings
- be honest: answer questions simply and truthfully and be prepared to say 'I don't know' rather than invent answers

- listen to what parents want, and always try to see the situation from their point of view.

More practical points at the time of death include:

- Allow the family to stay with the dead child for as long as they want.
- Explain that the child will get cold and change colour.
- Encourage the parents to wash and dress the child.
- If the child has to stay in hospital, reassure the parents they are welcome to return.

Parents also welcome the opportunity to visit the ward and talk to the nurses after the funeral.

Being informed about procedures following a death and the options available to parents is essential, and every ward should be equipped with a written protocol for staff and information leaflets for parents.

Midwives

Involvement

The status of the midwife gives her a special kind of authority and significance for parents. She may well be the first to discover or confirm the loss of a fetal heartbeat. She will be involved with late miscarriages and the delivery of a baby who has died *in utero*, and with a stillbirth of a previously well baby who suffers birth complications. Anticipated stillbirths tend to be the responsibility of senior midwives. In the event of an early cot death, the community midwife may still be visiting the mother before handing over to the health visitor.

Function

The midwife has a key role to play in the management of perinatal death and support of the parents. She works in partnership with the mother and consultant, which gives her an interpretive role, balancing medical needs with parental wishes. She prepares the mother for what will happen and keeps her informed of what is happening. After stillbirth, the midwife has a vital part to play in helping the parents to face the reality of the death. This includes the now standard procedures of taking photographs, handprints, and encouraging the parents to touch and hold the baby. It is also a listening role, giving permission to the parents to express feelings. Midwives who recognize the importance of parents seeing their malformed baby have discovered the reassurance this provides. They will find beauty in their baby somewhere, and without this opportunity will see a monster in their minds.

Fathers have traditionally been excluded from this kind of care, and may need encouragement – perhaps from a male staff member – to take advantage of the opportunities to see and handle the dead baby. Fathers who do not wish to see the baby may need help to understand the importance of this ritual for the mother.

On a practical level, the midwife is well placed to explain all the procedures to parents regarding registration, post-mortem and funeral arrangements.

Concerns

As midwifery is about being productive, the death of a baby represents total failure. The midwife will experience her own grief, guilt and anger, which means dealing with her own feelings as well as those of the parents.

The loss of a twin presents a very difficult situation. The tendency is to encourage the parents to concentrate on their joy for the live birth, but if they do not grieve for the dead one, problems arise about rejecting the surviving twin.

In hospitals without separate rooms for grieving parents, it is a dilemma whether to care for them on a ward with babies, or on a ward with no babies. Once the mother is discharged home, the caring midwife may be left anxious about continuing support.

Good practice

Much work has been done in recent years to implement the recommen- dations and guidelines published by the Stillbirth and Neonatal Death Society (SANDS). These emphasize the importance of giving parents information, choices and time to make their own decisions. Parents often do not know what is possible. Decisions in which parents should be involved include the following.

- Whether and when the mother should be induced when the baby has died in the womb.
- Whether and when life-support is withdrawn if the baby is born alive but known to be dying.
- Whether to see, hold, wash and dress the dead baby.
- Whether to have a post-mortem.
- Whether to take the baby home.
- How long the mother stays in hospital.

Involving fathers, and sometimes siblings or grandparents, is now the norm in most up-to-date maternity units. Millie and Derek, whose son Ben was stillborn, will always be grateful to their midwife for her patience and sensitivity:

'When she first asked us if we wanted to see him, we said no – we were feeling so tired and wretched. The next day she asked us again, but I was frightened what he would look like, and Derek didn't want me to get more upset. When my mum came the midwife asked if she wanted to see the baby, which she did, and then that gave us the courage to see him. She brought him in to us, and we held him and cried together and felt like a proper family.'

In the absence of a birth or death certificate, some hospitals issue their own 'certificates' to acknowledge the baby's life. Most maternity units now have a written protocol, which gives priority to parents' wishes, and many now have a separate room or suite where both parents can sleep over to spend time privately with their baby.

An experienced midwife adds a word of caution about checklists: 'They can't tell you what to say. You have to treat everyone as an individual and be sensitive to their needs.'

Police

Involvement

Child deaths involving the police are all sudden and traumatic: accidents, murders, suicides and cot deaths. They involve the police officer in unwelcome tasks, and require behaving with great tact, dignity and compassion. The inability to rescue a child from a house fire is reported to be particularly harrowing, as indeed it is for firefighters.

Function

It is the police function to report to the coroner any sudden death where the deceased has not been seen by a doctor in the previous month, or if the cause of death is uncertain. This is not generally appreciated, so the involvement of the police in the event of a cot death has to be explained carefully. The investigating officer's task is to enquire into the circumstances of the death, view the body and have the child identified prior to hospitalization for post-mortem. The removal of bedding and clothing to help with the pathologist's report needs to be handled with sensitivity.

'Giving the death message' is a police term for delivering news that a death has occurred, and is considered harder than dealing with the victim of an accident. The unexpected police officer knocking at the door is the stereotypical dread of all parents.

Where criminal investigations are concerned, ongoing contact with the family to keep them fully informed is not always seen as a priority for the police, but is vital to the parents.

Concerns

Delivering news of a child's death causes great anxiety about what to say and the reactions of the parents. Shifting attitudes away from the 'stiff upper lip' have brought a recognition of the distress and need to debrief afterwards with a senior or welfare officer.

Being asked for details of traumatic deaths is also stressful, with uncertainty about how much to say. There is a natural wish to protect parents, especially the mother, from unpleasant facts, and an inclination to defer to another person or later time. This can leave parents frustrated and resentful.

Seeking help for stress can be seen as a sign of weakness, with concerns about confidentiality if ongoing support is required to cope with personal reactions.

Good practice

Police forces all over the country are now recognizing the importance of preparing officers for these traumatic situations, with sessions of 'breaking bad news' and 'talking to parents' being included in training programmes. A traffic division on Merseyside enlisted the help of the Alder Centre to use the feedback of bereaved parents. Their experiences underline the importance of the following.

- Avoid protecting parents: they need to see and to know in order to grieve.
- Answer questions as honestly as possible.
- Involve both parents and keep the family together.
- Treat the family as you would like your own to be dealt with in similar circumstances.
- Wear plain clothes in sensitive situations, such as home visits after a cot death.
- Give parents time with their child: do not hurry them.
- Always refer to the child or baby by name.

Being well-informed helps. The officer feels more confident and the family reassured if they are clear about legal requirements, post-mortem and inquest procedures. The Foundation for the Study of Infant Deaths and the Scottish Cot Death Trust publish excellent information leaflets for police officers.

Every force has a designated person who takes on a welfare role. Northants Police Welfare officer, Elizabeth Grayson, is a trained counsellor who has organized a system of peer counsellors all over the county, ranging from cleaner to chief inspector. She says: 'When you deal with a child death, you must talk about it, and how you feel, to *someone*.'

Registrars of births, marriages and deaths

Involvement

The registrar of a medium-sized town (population 150 000) can expect to deal with one or two deaths of children per month, more if the local hospital has a maternity department. As the death must be registered in the district where it occurred, register offices in cities containing a paediatric hospital will have a much higher incidence. In busy offices, parents may have to wait a long time in a queue, perhaps having battled through a couple of wedding parties to get there. Some registrars go out to maternity hospitals to register births, stillbirths and neonatal deaths – a much appreciated service.

Function

The role of the registrar is to perform the legal requirement of recording information about the death, including data for statistics, and administering the paperwork relating to the disposal of the body. In this sense the registrar is accountable to the relevant government department – the general register office. The legislation concerning who can register, and where the registration takes place, does not allow for a mobile population. As one county service manager put it: 'We are managing a sevice in the 1990s with a framework developed in the 1830s.'

Concerns

The main concern is getting the registration done while parents are in distress. Spelling out the details of the child's death and seeing them recorded in black and white for the first time can be a gruelling experience for parents, and the registrar has to guide them through the form-filling in an emotionally charged atmosphere.

Amazingly, there is at present no statutory training for registrars, and therefore no preparation for dealing with bereaved relatives. However, a national working party is looking at introducing a national certificate of competence. Meanwhile, individual registrars already define good practice as putting people before paperwork.

Good practice

As defined by a parent:

'We went together to register Barry's death. There were several people waiting but the receptionist showed us to a small private room till the registrar was ready to see us. He was very courteous – said he was sorry about the reason for coming, and explained what had to be done. When Susan got upset, he put his pen down and waited till we were ready to go on. He checked he'd got all the details right, then gave us two copies of the death certificate. It may seem a little thing, but it was pleasing to see such nice handwriting.'

A registrar's comments:

'It's important to explain clearly to parents what my task is, and then I try to ask the questions as sensitively as possible. For example, I have to ask whether the informant was present at the death. The bureaucratic version is: "Were you present at the death?" But I prefer to ask: "Were you able to be present at the death?", which takes into account their experience in a more human way. I make a point of using the baby's or child's name as often as possible, as a mark of respect.'

Social workers

Involvement

Fieldworkers will meet child death only rarely, when the affected family is already being supported or where a child is subject to child protection procedures.

The hospital social worker will be closely involved as part of the care team in both acute and ongoing situations, and may be the one person who remains constant to the family throughout the treatment process.

Function

The hospital social worker's primary role is to support the family and to be an advocate for the parents. This support is available to all families, regardless of status, and facilitates communication between patient, parents and staff. Advocacy means representing the parents' wishes and concerns, and acting as an interpreter and mediator; it requires good counselling skills. The counselling function can continue well into the first year of bereavement and beyond, with home visits and facilitating group support.

Practical support includes providing information about benefits and entitlements during terminal illness, helping with transport and family care at the time of the death and guiding the parents through the first days of bereavement. As well as providing information about legalities, the social worker is ideally placed to help the parents make informed choices about the funeral and to consider the needs of other family members. There may be some overlap here with the midwife, health visitor or community nurse, depending on existing relationships, making good communication essential and maybe indicating a co-ordinating role with other professionals and agencies.

Concerns

Those who have opted to work in areas with a high incidence of mortality, such as casualty or intensive care, are vulnerable to accumulated stress and need well-developed support and supervision systems. Operating as a buffer between families and professionals can also be very taxing.

Child protection social workers are faced with acute dilemmas and anxieties when the life of a child is thought to be at risk. When a child dies as a result of neglect or abuse, the professional is left with feelings of anger, helplessness and guilt, and needs intense support.

Good practice

Social workers in the hospital setting have to be willing to undertake bereavement work, be aware of the effects of grief for themselves and others, and be prepared to work in a multidisciplinary way. A commitment to the rights of parents and the advocacy role underpins all good practice. One maternity unit social worker comments:

> 'I aim to work towards parents feeling that everything that could be done, was done, and that they may be left with as few regrets as possible. If they can say this, it makes their grieving easier.'

Counselling skills are basic to all social work, although the level of sensitivity needed for this emotive area indicates the benefits of further training. In order to use these skills effectively, there needs to be an acceptance within their management structure that bereavement support is part of good working practice.

Above all, the social worker is valued by parents as a good listener and as someone who can reduce their isolation. When Jo's baby David died, the GP gave them the telephone number of an Alder Hey social worker:

> 'This was my first glimmer of hope ... and I clutched that 'phone number for two weeks before making contact. She just let us talk. She introduced us to a support group of bereaved parents. They too carried a big ball of black pain around – what a relief it was to meet them.'

Teachers

Involvement

The whole school community is deeply affected when a pupil dies, and teachers are indirectly involved when a pupil's sibling or young friend dies. The staff of specialist schools for children with life-threatening conditions include physiotherapists, occupational therapists and domestic personnel as well as teachers. Hospital teachers form significant relationships with children who are terminally ill.

Function

The class teacher forms an important link between school and family when a child is hospitalized, keeping the child in touch with peers and the normality of school life. When the child dies, teachers provide models for pupils in how they react. A senior teacher may well take the lead in liaising with parents, formally acknowledging the death in school, and facilitating some ceremony or ritual to express the school's mourning. Practical tasks include amending class lists and collecting anything belonging to the child.

In the case of sudden death, teachers will have more extreme reactions to deal with as shockwaves run through the school, causing anger and anxiety.

Bereaved siblings present teachers with another challenge of what to say and how to accommodate their grief. Trusted teachers may be required to act as a counsellor and confidante for the child, or even for the parents. In the rare cases when more is required, the teacher is ideally placed to monitor the reactions of the grieving child, alert the parents and enlist specialist help.

Concerns

The effects of a teenage suicide are particularly traumatic and teachers may be concerned about aroused curiosity and copy-cat attempts. In fact, any cloak of silence increases the students' anxiety. Fears of hysterical reactions may also smother open acknowledgement of any sudden death.

A death that occurs during holidays presents special problems as to how to handle the news on return to school. If a death occurs on a school trip or organized educational holiday, when teachers are *in loco parentis*, extensive debriefing and counselling will be required.

Teachers are not always informed that a pupil has lost a sibling, which makes it difficult to respond appropriately to any problematic reactions.

Good practice

Any school that exposes students to death as a natural part of life, through nature studies, biology, personal and social education programmes, will be better placed to deal openly with the unnatural death of a child. Many secondary schools now include 'death studies' on the pastoral curriculum, and devote some in-service training time to preparing teachers by looking at their own attitudes to death. Younger children may need help with the difference between death and sleep, and are able to cope better with clear, unambiguous answers to questions. Many good books are now on the market for all ages to help children make sense of their experience.

In practical terms, the eventuality of child death should be included in the school protocol, with clear guidelines as to who does what. Acknowledging the death is always important. Teachers should keep any of the child's work for parents to collect, if they so wish.

Head teachers, or those with special responsibility for pastoral care, need to consider ways and means of communicating information about a dying child, or the death of a child, which will impact on their pupils. While confidentiality has to be respected, good liaison with parents and the school health service or community paediatrician will make it easier to confront such a sensitive situation.

A primary school teacher offers the benefit of her experience in the loss of a pupil who died from leukaemia:

'When he returned to school after his transplant, I tried to treat him as normally as possible. At the same time, I kept in close contact with the parents, and the children helped to organize a sponsored swim for leukaemia research. They wrote to him and visited during his last illness. When he died, the children were told in a calm and honest way. Many of us cried and I felt it important that I did not hide my grief.'

A senior secondary teacher offers this advice to colleagues:

'Never underestimate pupils' feelings, as siblings or friends, and don't underestimate your own influence for good. Listen to them, and try to understand beyond the words: they may ask for your help in a roundabout way. It takes courage.'

4 Guidelines for all

Sensitivity and compassion are developed rather than taught, but there are some general principles that supply the helper with more confidence, and there are skills that can be practised. The importance of support for the helper cannot be overstated, and the purpose of supervision will be discussed. Training needs are covered by the suggested contents of a training programme, including awareness raising, listening skills and some helping strategies. Finally, all readers are invited to address themselves to the resources questionnaire at the end of the chapter.

General principles

Regardless of role or situation, the most basic principle is the importance of *listening to what individual people say they want rather than presuming what they need*. After that, it is useful to bear in mind the themes that run through the experience of families quoted in this book. Families say they want: information, choices, control and permission to grieve.

The following principles have emerged from the experience of the first three years of the Alder Centre.

Being there is more important than what you do; listening is more important than talking

There is often a pressure to know the right things to say, and a fear of saying the wrong things. We can end up feeling so anxious that we cannot listen! Be assured that simply by being in attendance or by making your visit you are doing something useful. If you are offering emotional support by listening as well, then you are doing a great deal. You are conveying the messages that the family is *not* carrying a social disease and that you are not afraid of their pain. You are still going to feel pretty helpless, but it is important to recognize that as a feature of bereavement support, and not to let the feelings of helplessness prevent your making contact. More about attending and listening skills can be found on pages 78–9.

Be clear about your involvement

First, you need to be clear about your role and what support you are offering. This should then be made clear to the bereaved person, even if your professional title appears to make it obvious. Are you there as part of your job, or out of personal concern? Are you representing an agency? Is this a one-off contact or are you offering ongoing care? Are you offering practical or emotional support? At the outset, a named introduction is a common courtesy, and it is good practice to leave behind some written confirmation of who you are and where you can be contacted.

These may well be routine procedures, but they take on added importance in bereavement when people commonly feel impotent and confused. The newly bereaved may be particularly vulnerable to people who are keen to peddle their own belief systems. Remember, too, that many bereaved parents lose faith in any justice in the world and are sensitive to further disappointment. The helper therefore needs to be scrupulous about keeping appointments, keeping time and promising only what is realistic in terms of further support.

The issue of confidentiality also needs to be considered carefully. Reassurance should be given that private information will be treated sensitively, and that any information shared is strictly in the interests of the bereaved person. Sort out with your supervisor the conditions, if any, that would compromise confidentiality.

Use the child's name

This means so much to parents, for the name keeps alive the memory of this child. It is an acknowledgement that the child really existed at a time when it is difficult for parents to separate reality from fantasy. Saying the name also means that you are interested in the child, whether or not you knew him, and that you recognize the meaning of the child's absence. It can be tempting to tiptoe round the child, in the mistaken belief that mentioning him will upset the parent. A moment's reflection is sufficient to realize that the grief for the child is ever-present, that being 'upset' is entirely appropriate and that it is our own fear of painful feelings getting in the way. Asking about the child, looking at photographs and mementoes are ways of paying respect to child and parent, and help to facilitate expression of grief.

Avoid platitudes and euphemisms

Having respect for another person, regardless of age, race and social background, is one of the core conditions for a helping relationship. Respect can be shown for the other person's feelings, thoughts and beliefs, whether or not one agrees with them. Lack of respect is shown in patronizing comments, discounting remarks, moralizing and platitudes.

A platitude is defined as 'an empty remark made as if it were important'. To apply well-worn phrases which so easily miss the mark is insulting. Using any phrase which begins 'At least . . .' only serves to undermine the bereaved person's suffering. Sadly parents hear them all too often: 'At least you have two other healthy children' or 'At least you are young enough to have another child'.

A euphemism is a device for describing something unpleasant in milder terms in an attempt to avoid the unpleasantness. Death is riddled with euphemisms such as 'We've lost him' and 'He passed away'. It has already been pointed out how mischievous such phrases can be for children, and that their persistent use may indicate continuing denial of the reality of the death. Euphemisms should not be used by carers and helpers because they can cause misunderstanding and because they avoid reality. There is no way of dressing up the harsh fact of death.

Each bereavement is unique

First, it helps to remember that each child is a unique individual. Even a premature baby will have unique characteristics. All the particular features of the child need to be mourned, and as the child is often idealized by the parents, which is not to deny the special courage of many terminally ill children, you may be able to help them grieve for the whole child, warts and all.

Second, it is important to recognize each bereaved person as an individual and to allow them the uniqueness of their own loss without constant comparisons with others' experiences or, worse still, your own. This denies the bereaved person the opportunity to be seen and accepted for herself. Out of this attention to the individual comes the ability to see more clearly the world through her eyes. Empathy is another of the core conditions which encourage trust in a helping relationship.

People come before theory. An understanding of patterns and common features is valuable: it serves to reassure you, and shared experience is comforting for the bereaved. But you can never presume to know how it is, so avoid saying, 'I know how you feel'.

It is also useful to remember that everything has to be done again by the parents and family for the first time after the child's death – the first meal, the first visit to a supermarket, the first Christmas, the first holiday.

Seeing is believing

It is difficult to accept the reality of death, and more so if a healthy child dies suddenly. Those who grieve a personal loss need to see some evidence to connect what they understand in their heads with what they know in their hearts. Parents want to say goodbye and feel physically close in death. Parents have the right to see their dead child, however shocking or distressing that may be. They need preparation more than protection. Your patient understanding may be required in helping them consider the pros and cons, with time to make an informed choice (*see* Chapter 1, pages 9–11; Chapter 3, pages 63–4; Chapter 5, pages 89–92).

The same general principle applies to whether siblings should be encouraged or discouraged to see the dead child. Children are often resentful later if they were not given the choice. Very often, children are protected from knowing the full extent of the last illness and from seeing the dying child in the last hours. Even children of a very young age benefit from being included in the reality of the situation. These sensitive issues are for the parents to resolve, but they may ask for your help in thinking them through.

Fantasy is worse than reality

Knowledge is power, and having information gives one a greater sense of control in any situation. When parental responsibility is involved, the need for information is paramount. The paternalism of the medical profession is thankfully giving way to an understanding of how important it is to keep parents fully involved and consulted. As well as being ethically correct, this enables parents to work through their reactions to the death. What is not known will be imagined, and almost invariably the fantasy turns out to be worse than the reality. Younger children have the doubtful advantage of literal imagination, which can be very confusing and worrying for them if they hear only half a story and if questions are not answered honestly.

Involve all the family

At the time of the death the mother is often protected from harsh realities, but afterwards she tends to be the focus of attention: ask directly after the welfare of the father and other children too. If your advice and help are sought in the practical arrangements for the funeral and other rituals, remember the benefits if all the family can be involved. Parents, children and grandparents are much more likely to be able to support each other in their grief later if they have felt included in decisions about the form of service, the wording on a wreath or headstone, and what happens to the child's possessions.

There are no experts

Of course there are those who have more experience of dealing with child death and bereaved families, and those whose training equips them for special tasks. But in most situations the person best qualified to offer support is someone who is already known and trusted by the family. Bereavement work makes everyone feel inadequate and it is tempting to look around for an 'expert' who can do a better job. The only experts on this unique experience are the family. Being supportive is much more about being there, rather than doing something. You will, however, need support and supervision for a variety of reasons.

You will need support

If you were involved with the child's care before the death or at the time of death, you will need some outlet for your own reactions. Feelings of failure and helplessness need to be expressed without fear of being judged as inadequate. Sensitive support of bereaved families is stressful and requires recognition of the demands being made of you. You may find yourself affected on several levels: by the family's grief, by memories of your own losses, by fears for the future, by anger and frustration at feeling so powerless to help. *If these feelings are not safely discharged, you either risk your own mental health or compromise your capacity for compassion.* You may be lucky enough to have instant support available amongst colleagues, but if you are working in isolation it is essential to have time built into your work schedule to offload. This may be combined with supervision from someone responsible for overseeing your work (*see* below).

The learning points from these general principles are now summarized and offered as a check against your own experience:

- show your concern by being there for the family
- listen more than you talk
- be clear about what you are offering
- be courteous and considerate
- use the child's name
- encourage the family to talk about the child
- avoid meaningless platitudes
- respect the uniqueness of the family's experience
- enable the family to make informed choices
- pay attention to brothers and sisters
- encourage the family to share decisions
- do not underestimate the value of your support
- get support for yourself.

Supervision

Supervision means different things to different professionals. It can be used for quality control, time management, evaluation and support.

In the context of bereavement, the supervisory role might be better described as consultation, and it is essential to good practice.

Why is supervision so important?

- Being so close to death is stressful. When the death is that of a child, and when the death is sudden, the added dimensions of tragedy and trauma make this a very difficult area of work.
- Working with death and bereavement tends to be isolating, reflecting the lonely experience of grief itself.
- Supporting someone in grief can cause a blurring of personal and professional boundaries.
- Child death increasingly involves litigation issues.

What are the functions of supervision?

Support
Stress is alleviated by sharing the feelings of sadness, helplessness and inadequacy that arise. Having these feelings acknowledged prevents isolation. It also helps to have your skills affirmed and your efforts valued.

Clarification
Your role and level of involvement need to be clarified for your own sake, as well as that of the bereaved person. Being clear about your task and adjusting it to the needs of the person prevents you from becoming overinvolved. You also need to know where you stand regarding any policy or practice guidelines operated by your department or agency. Ethical issues that need addressing include questions about confidentiality and contact with other agencies.

Co-ordination
Supervision is the ideal forum for seeing your work in a wider context of various kinds of support for the family, encouraging co-operation and the marshalling of extra resources.

Evaluation
As well as providing on-going assessment of whether objectives are being met, supervision enables you to evaluate your skills, experience and training needs. An objective view can be gained of your potential and your limitations.

Advice/consultation
This may relate to information about other resources, ideas for helping strategies and deliberations about whether to refer to another agency.

Protection

This again relates to the emotive nature of bereavement support and the drain on personal resources. Losses that occur in private life can affect professional attitudes and behaviour, and vice versa. Discussion of these affective factors helps to keep a sense of perspective.

Where can you get supervision?

If bereavement support forms a major part of your work, you should have regular, individual supervision with someone who has experience in this field and is familiar with the issues. That person could be your line manager, or you may need an external supervisor for your bereavement work.

Some of the supervisory functions listed above can be performed in a supervision group. Such a group can be made up of colleagues within the same work setting, or it can have a multidisciplinary membership of professionals concerned with similar issues.

If bereavement work is only occasional, you need to identify someone to whom you can go for short-term support and consultation.

Training

There is a strong case to be argued for loss and bereavement issues to be included on any basic training course in the health and caring professions, so that everyone has an opportunity to prepare themselves mentally. Specialist short courses follow more naturally when some experience has been acquired.

The starting point for any training input is raising awareness of the personal anxieties that threaten to get in the way of dealing compassionately with others. The taboos associated with death in the Western world can be challenged only by confronting our fears and prejudices.

Awareness

Reflecting on our own losses enables us to:

- identify reactions and ways of coping which give insights into others' experiences
- recognize areas of loss that have been difficult to resolve
- realize that working with someone grieving similar loss will trigger associated reactions to our past and feared losses
- acknowledge the difficulty of dealing with death in terms of our own mortality.

Acknowledging concerns that commonly beset those who support the bereaved is a reassuring exercise. Such concerns include:

- how will I cope?
- will I get sucked into others' distress?
- I won't know what to say or do
- should I show my feelings?

Acknowledgement of our own limitations helps to make these anxieties more manageable. A sense of vocation is associated with professions that seek to heal, empower, develop and support other people. It is therefore important to be prepared for the following feelings:

- feeling powerless to help
- a sense of failure and even guilt
- being inadequate for the task.

These reactions belong to the nature of grief. They do not deny the value of your support and care.

Skills

The two foundation skills required for bereavement support are basic to all effective communication: attending and listening. They are, of course, interrelated. Both sound simple but can be extremely difficult in practice, particularly when dealing with painful feelings. The learning points summarized below are best made by setting up exercises that allow participants to experience the effects of good and bad practice.

Attending

Paying attention means being alert to someone and being interested in what they have to say, which communicates the message that they are of value. That in itself encourages trust and free expression, and has a healing effect. Attending means suspending one's own concerns and prejudices, and being in a state of 'not knowing'. As well as conveying respect, attending also enables the listener to observe the whole person as communicated by body language and non-verbal behaviour. Good attention is demonstrated by:

- setting the scene: even before the communication starts, the way in which a person is greeted conveys respect
- making eye-contact is crucial; facial expressions, nods and grunts also provide physical evidence of being attended to
- removing barriers such as desks, equipment and papers, and sitting at the same level
- avoiding distracters such as bleeps and telephones.

Listening

Listening is a complex activity. It includes:

- giving attention
- receiving information
- taking in the thoughts and feelings conveyed
- interpreting behaviour
- noticing key points and themes
- checking that you have heard and understood correctly.

The focus remains on the speaker when the listener reflects back what has been heard. Restatements, paraphrasing and summarizing the messages received form an important part of the process for several reasons:

- the speaker is assured of your understanding
- if you have got it wrong, the speaker can correct you
- the speaker can hear the effect of what she is saying.

Listening involves considerable self-discipline. It means suspending your own assumptions, judgements, advice and solutions. It may also mean tolerating silence, allowing the speaker time and space to gather thoughts and give expression to feelings.

Helping strategies

While active listening forms the cornerstone of bereavement support, to facilitate the expression of the disordered thoughts and feelings of grief, other approaches may be required for ongoing support. More directive strategies may also be indicated when the bereaved person finds it difficult to talk, or when uncompleted mourning tasks have been identified.

Most of the ideas that follow are simple but can be powerfully effective. A training event is the ideal opportunity to try them out on yourself and colleagues.

Prompts

Some people welcome invitations to talk about their loved one, particularly if they have been discouraged from doing so by others. Open questions about the child might be:

'Can you tell me more about . . .?'

'What sort of child was he?'

'What are your special memories?'

Photographs and mementoes provide a fund of recollections, and a genuine interest in sharing them encourages warmth and trust.

Linking

One of the tasks of mourning is making sense of what has happened, and finding a place for the loss which offers some meaning. The bereaved may need some help in linking the past to the present, and this can be done by talking them through the process of change, perhaps over three meetings.

1. Invite reminiscences of what life was like before the child died – a typical weekday, holiday and so on – for self and family.
2. Ask for a (repeat) rehearsal of the events at the time of the child's death.
3. Invite reflections on how life has changed after the child died, and how things are different now.

Rituals

Bereavement is made up of many little goodbyes, and it may be appropriate to construct together some private rituals to help the bereaved deal with difficult memories. For instance, a parent at the Alder Centre requested help with revisiting the road junction where her daughter had been killed years previously. Another parent helped her child grieve for a friend, whose funeral they had been unable to attend, by releasing helium balloons with goodbye messages on them.

Writing

For many parents and siblings, writing becomes an important therapeutic tool. When such writing can be shared, it is a powerful communicator of inner feelings.

For those who are anguished by things left unsaid to the child, the device of writing a letter, addressed as it were to the child, can be liberating. Alternatively an audio tape could be made, with messages interspersed with favourite music.

Drawing

Children are less inhibited about drawing than adults, and may derive greater benefit from pictures than words. Images and colours help to give shape to memories and complex emotions.

Scrapbooks

This is another useful approach with children, but is equally valuable to adults, and a great activity to include all the family, or the child's schoolfriends. Photographs, keepsakes, written memories, pictures of favourite pop stars and activities can all contribute to a shared album of memories. This may be a useful suggestion when one of the family is left with an impossibly idealized picture of the child, as the scrapbook can easily accommodate different images – the comic and the naughty as well as the sad and the good.

Geneogram

This is a diagrammatic way of depicting the family, like a family tree, which records births, marriages and deaths and provides a tool for exploring family relationships. It is drawn up with the help of the bereaved, and is useful for gaining a wider perspective on the significance of the child's death for different family members.

Resources questionnaire

All readers are invited to assess their resources and needs by considering these questions.

1. How does my personal experience affect my attitude to bereavement?

2. What is the level of awareness of my own actual and feared losses?

3. Can I identify the other person's needs, and the tasks involved in my support?

4. What is my role?

5. What relevant skills do I have?

6. How do I recognize my limitations? Am I being honest, or modest?

7. Do I have training needs?

8. Do I know when, how and where to refer on for more specialist help?

9. Are my needs for consultation and support being met?

5 Guidelines for stressful situations

There are certain key situations when the words, actions and attitudes of professionals can have a lasting impact on the family, for good or ill. Advice may be sought by parents who are emotionally vulnerable. Others may be temporarily hostile towards those who seek to help them. Years later, parents tend to remember with utmost clarity the detail of turning points in their child's illness and treatment. And in the heightened sensitivity of their grief, thoughtless comments add to their pain just as caring gestures are treasured.

Knowing this adds to the sense of heavy responsibility at such times for professionals to 'get it right' or at least avoid 'putting one's foot in it'. Anxiety is a natural response when faced with painful emotions and a sense of helplessness. There are no blueprints for any given situation, but some general guidelines can provide signposts.

It needs to be stressed that each situation is unique and people's reactions are unpredictable. No-one can get it right all the time, but the sincerity of trying to do one's best is what matters.

Breaking bad news

One father recalls how much it meant to him that when his son died the doctor was visibly upset at the bedside. By contrast, one mother is still outraged, 10 years later, that the doctor yawned after telling her that her daughter had just died. Another mother remembers: 'We held her until the Sister said "she's gone now", and I hated her so much I could have done murder − but I know I needed to hear the words to believe it.' The task of communicating bad news is unenviable, whether at the time of diagnosis, treatment results, accident, post-mortem results or inquest. It gives rise to similar reactions as experienced when being on the receiving end: anxiety, fear, panic, anger, helplessness, failure, sadness, despair. Some of the anxiety may be about the other person's reactions, because the bearers of bad news have been known to be lynched! The message-carrier is certainly an easy target for first reactions of angry disbelief, particularly as a member of the medical profession.

A simple checklist is offered below to help identify the ideal circumstances for breaking bad news.

Why?

This may seem obvious, but the underlying question is an ethical one and raises issues of information and control. Is the amount of information given on a 'need-to-know' or 'right-to-know' basis? Nothing enrages parents more than discovering later that information about their own child has been withheld.

When?

The answer to the above will determine the timing. On a 'right-to-know' basis, the guideline must be: as soon as possible.

By whom?

Qualities are favoured more than position: ideally it should be someone known and trusted, who shows sensitivity and has good communication skills. Most parents say it helps if the person has a continuing involvement with them, rather than someone who appears and then disappears. The importance of the authority of the person seems to depend on the nature of the information. A complex diagnosis, for example, requires specialist knowledge to answer parents' questions. In other hospital situations, the nursing staff offer more continuity.

Where?

Parents invariably recall the setting, and there is a strong association with the room and the importance of the occasion. The place should be somewhere comfortable, private and without interruption.

How?

If at all possible, the breaking of bad news should be in a face-to-face situation, and it is important to look the person in the eye. Take a few minutes before going into the situation to check your demeanour and gather your thoughts. If a telephone call is unavoidable, due consideration needs to be given to the likely impact of shock and distress.

Every effort should be made to tell both parents together. If this is not possible, another family member or friend should be present for support.

The message should be unambiguous to avoid misunderstanding, and questions should be answered as honestly as possible. Euphemisms are not helpful. In the case of giving a diagnosis of terminal illness, a balance needs to be struck between realism and hope.

Shock and disbelief may require time for the information to be received, so it is important to go at their pace. This means checking out their understanding of what you have said, and repeating or restating the information as necessary.

Check their responses: ask how they are feeling, what are their immediate concerns, are there any questions they want to ask. Some people react to bad news with denial, apparent apathy or by trivializing it, and these defences need to be respected. Before leaving the interview, ongoing support and follow-up needs to be ensured. This may involve transport arrangements, medical attention, alerting local resources and providing reassurance that there will be opportunities for addressing questions and concerns at a future time.

Finally, you will need the support of a colleague, ideally to accompany you or at least to debrief you afterwards.

Some experiences of parents

'Christine had various tests at the hospital, but we weren't told what they were for. Then one day we had a letter informing us that Christine had been diagnosed as a cystic fibrosis child and we were to visit the clinic in three weeks' time. We had no idea what cystic fibrosis was. A friend gave us the address of the Cystic Fibrosis Fund and we sent off for some leaflets.'

'We pinned all our hopes on Jason having this operation to remove the tumour. He seemed to recover very well, but the consultant was doubtful. Then Jason went downhill fast, and in the end the consultant sat down with us and said there was nothing more they could do for him. We'd got to know him quite well and it was like we were all in this together. He answered all our questions and we looked at the options. He taped that session and gave us the tape to take home: it was a great help to go over it again and play it to our parents. You can't remember half of what's said otherwise.'

'Tracy lived for 11 days. I'm usually squeamish about illness and medical things, but I wanted to know every detail about her condition. The doctor went through the post-mortem and answered all my questions as best she could – she was honest about not knowing all the answers – but it was so important for me to know all there was to know. My mum came with me, which was a help.'

'The police officer who called said that the paramedics had taken Simon to hospital and there was still hope of reviving him. It wasn't till we got to the hospital two hours later that we discovered he was dead when they found him. We felt so resentful about that lie. Did the policeman think he was doing us a favour? Our son was dead for over two hours and other people knew it and we didn't. The hospital doctor who confirmed the death was cold and detached. We wished he had shown some feeling, at least said he was sorry.'

Emergency procedures and intensive care

'We recognize that relatives have a part to play in our work, and that we help to create memories which will affect them for the rest of their lives.' So says the clinical nurse specialist at the accident and emergency department of Wythenshawe Hospital, Manchester, where the consultant and casualty team follow an enlightened policy that allows parents to be involved and fully informed throughout treatment. Lack of information and involvement are the most consistent regrets and resentments of parents of children receiving emergency medical care.

Traditionally the care of relatives of the patient has been seen as a nursing issue, as death is not a medical problem. However, more and more consultants have a growing understanding of bereavement support as part of the total health care package. At Alder Hey Children's Hospital in Liverpool, the prevailing philosophy is that the family is the patient, not just the child. Given this commitment, traditional objections to involving the family can be faced and overcome. More hospitals in the UK now operate open access to parents, which means they need never be separated from their child.

Protocol

The unpredictability of an emergency makes it impossible to lay down any set protocol for dealing with relatives, whose reactions are not consistent. The family's trauma is matched by the frantic efforts of the staff to save the child's life. Some parents merely wish to be reassured that something is being done, while others want to be present to see exactly what is going on. However, some general principles will guide good practice for the benefit of parents and help staff deal better with the feelings of failure when a child dies.

Teamwork

The staff team, from cleaner to consultant, will need to work through their own feelings and reactions in order to adopt a team approach. The team may also include the chaplain and social worker. Good team relationships are essential to the kind of flexibility and communication required.

Identified person

Someone on the team needs to be allocated to the care of the parents, to explain what is happening and to facilitate their needs short of obstructing treatment. Parents need to be prepared and cautioned about what they will see. When parents do not wish to be present during treatment, they will need to be kept closely informed. The identified person may be allocated by role: it may be the social worker or chaplain who routinely acts as parental support. A medically-trained person may be thought more appropriate for answering questions and explaining treatment procedures. At Wythenshawe it could be any one of the team, but is usually the consultant or sister. They argue that if relatives are given high enough priority, existing staff can be used without compromising patients' care.

Resuscitation

The attendance of parents during resuscitation is a contentious issue, and professional misgivings have to be challenged as well as respected. Common objections are:

- staff feel inhibited
- parents need protecting from seeing aggressive treatment
- parents get in the way
- staff are vulnerable to criticism.

These fears stem from being faced with other people's acute emotions and the defences which are erected to cope with one's own feelings. These *can* be confronted successfully once the right of parents to attend, if they wish, is accepted. In practice, the staff at Wythenshawe have met few problems. They have found that parents who attend resuscitation are more concerned with the child than the treatment.

An implication is whether parents can then be involved in the decision about when resuscitation efforts should cease, always a difficult time for staff. If, when all hope has long gone, parents are unable to face the reality, the consultant has to take professional responsibility for the decision.

There are some situations where the decision to withdraw life-support is fraught with difficulty. After accident-related trauma, certain criteria to establish brain stem death have to be met, which may entail necessary delay before the life support machine can be switched off. This demands particular sensitivity in explaining the situation to parents.

For most parents, being there at the moment of death and being able to touch or hold the child are essential to feeling they did all they could, that the child was not alone amongst strangers, and that they were able to let him go. All family members should have opportunity to say these goodbyes, including young siblings, as long as this is acceptable to the parents.

Practicalities

It is necessary to have a separate room for relatives, of course, but also important to have a private space where the parents can be with their child immediately after the death for as long as they wish. Their primary support person needs to be available to them during that time without pressure from colleagues to be elsewhere. Procedures and options need to be explained, with a written booklet for reference on leaving. Parents who find it difficult to leave the child may find comfort in leaving something personal with the body. It is much appreciated when staff handle and address the child with the same warmth and respect as before death.

After the death

This is a time when professionals who are correctly informed and aware of the issues can be very helpful to bereaved families. Parents who are plunged into grief will usually need the guidance of the nurse, doctor, social worker or chaplain, particularly when the death was unexpected. Even families who can draw on the experience of other bereavements are unlikely to feel confident of their rights and obligations when a child dies. Their need for advice and guidance is never greater than at this time, not to take control away from them, but so that they can make their own informed choices. The assumption should not be made, as it often is, that bereaved parents – especially the mother – are not in a fit state to make decisions.

Sudden death presents the biggest challenge. There has been no preparation and there is no continuity of care. The availability of hospital social workers and chaplains will be variable. Many hospital doctors see their role finishing with the death of the child, leaving follow-up care to nursing staff or to other professionals.

Roles and responsibilities need to be clear

The first and most important guideline, therefore, is to ensure adequate systems are in place, and that staff induction programmes make them known. Co-ordinated care avoids the 'rugby pass' type of management.

A designated person should be responsible for the on-going care of parents or for co-ordinating that initial support, in line with the Department of Health guidelines, *Care of the Dying in Hospital*.

The family's GP should be informed as soon as possible as the most obvious primary care co-ordinator in the community.

Giving advice and information

Information given to parents must be accurate and consistent, with an opportunity to talk it through rather than simply being offered it in written form.

Hospital staff should be aware of cultural and religious differences, with access to translators in case of language difficulties, and to signers for the deaf.

When decisions need to be made, parents should not be hurried to suit hospital routines, and time should always be allowed for parents to change their minds.

It helps to remember that the child continues to belong to the parents, except for the coroner's brief legal 'ownership' in the case of a post-mortem. For example, talking to parents about when they are 'allowed' to see their child denies their *right* to do so.

Practical examples of the kind of information required follow.

Legalities

By law a doctor must confirm the death.

The death is then registered with the registrar for births, marriages and deaths, by either or both parents, whether married or not, in the district where the death occurred. In extreme circumstances, someone else present at the death or during the last illness can do this. In the case of a newly-born baby, the birth must be registered first. The registrar issues:

- the death certificate, for which a small fee is payable
- a white BD8 form for the DSS
- a green disposal form, which is needed by the undertaker to remove the body from hospital.

However, the parents are entitled to remove the body themselves once a doctor has confirmed the cause of death. This situation may arise when the child dies after 5 pm and the parents are unwilling to leave the child in the hospital mortuary overnight or over the weekend before they can register the death. Parents have the right to know that this option is available to them, however undesirable this course of action may appear.

In cases of sudden death or where the cause of death is not known

- The doctor must inform the coroner.
- The coroner's officer, usually a police officer, will visit the hospital and/or home and interview parents.
- A post-mortem examination is normally required.
- Once a medical cause of death is established, the death can be registered and the body released.

Parents should be asked if they want to know what the post-mortem examination entails. Many do not like to ask, but are later filled with remorse for not knowing, and may suffer from fantasies of butchery. Reassurance of standard procedures and sensitive handling of the body are welcome.

In cases where a post-mortem is not legally required, it may still be requested for the sake of medical research, and is then a matter of choice. Post-mortems are forbidden to Muslims unless ordered by the coroner, and are problematic for Hindus.

Access to the child's body

It is essential that the parents are given privacy to spend as long as they wish with the child after death in hospital. It is helpful for one of the nursing staff to prepare them for the changes that will occur in the temperature and appearance of the body. They should be invited to take part in the washing and dressing of the child's body and other laying-out procedures, but should not be pressed to do so. Practising Muslim, Hindu and Jewish families are responsible for attending to the body to carry out traditional post-death rituals.

The taking of a photograph or lock of hair is now routinely offered by most hospitals, although the family's permission must be obtained: it is important to Muslims that the hair is not cut after death.

Parents are often very anxious to know where the child's body is taken after they have said their goodbyes. Again, they often do not like to ask: they are swept along in a personal nightmare and feel constrained by institutional procedures. They need to be told exactly what will happen to the child, where the body will be kept, who will tend to it and when they are able to visit. Ideally an 'open access' policy enables parents to come back to the hospital and spend time with their child at any hour of the day or night.

Options for where the child rests before the funeral

It is incumbent on professionals to make parents aware of the options, as some parents do not realize that they can have their child's body at home for some or all of the time before the funeral. Those families who have exercised this option have found it very beneficial. Again, it is a question of giving control back where it belongs.

Burial or cremation?

Parents naturally shrink from the thought of either burying or burning their child's body. Muslims are always buried, never cremated. All adult Hindus are cremated, but infants and young children may be buried. Orthodox Jews are always buried, but those of a more liberal persuasion may choose cremation. Where religious faith allows a choice, parents may welcome talking through the pros and cons with an objective outsider before making such an irrevocable decision. This means allowing time for making informed decisions. Having a specific place to visit is an important consideration for most families. An unforeseen dilemma can later occur when a grandparent or other relative generously offers to open an existing family grave so that the baby or child is not 'alone'. This may be an attractive idea at the time, but can be later regretted with the realization that the parents are then unable to join their child after death, as they would if they had opened a new family grave. These are Lisa's reflections:

'I was in such a daze after Carl died, but I knew I didn't want him buried. I couldn't have coped with the thought of his little body under the ground. There's a special garden of remembrance in our town where the ashes of babies can be scattered, so that's what we did. It seemed a nice idea to have him with other children. But I wish someone had told us that we could have bought a special little plot there. When we visit, I envy other parents who can plant flowers and have a little plaque to sit by.

Another thing I realized too late, after talking to other mums, was that I could have had Carl home before the funeral. They were very good at the hospital and let us visit him, and then we went to see him at the chapel of rest, but it was never long enough. I'd have liked him home for a least a couple of days.'

Funeral expenses

Funeral costs vary and it is advisable to obtain more than one quotation. Some funeral directors deliver a free basic service for any child who dies under the age of 16. Parents who can ill afford a funeral may reject this as charity, and need reassurance that a free service is of equal quality and is likely to indicate a particular sensitivity to child death situations. The hospital has an obligation to arrange and pay for the funeral of stillborn children, whether born in hospital or at home.

Families receiving Income Support or other DSS benefits are entitled to help with some or all of the funeral costs, and with the cost of transporting the body within the UK if the child dies away from home. The hospital social work department will help with the application to the Social Fund.

Attending the funeral

The funeral presents a ritual opportunity for family and community to say final goodbyes, and for others to pay their respects to the grieving family.

The advisability of young children attending funerals

Parents often consult professionals about whether their young children should go to the funeral. This is really a question of what adults can tolerate. Any temptation to tell parents what to do should be resisted. It is much more helpful to explore with them the pros and cons, to offer points of view they may not have considered, and encourage them to trust their own judgement. When parents are caught between their own instincts to take the children and the disapproving voices of older relatives, the task is one of reassurance.

Most children who were denied the opportunity to attend a sibling's funeral later regret this. Those who would not have wished to go regret not being given the choice. The age at which children can be trusted with such a choice will depend on the degree of openness in the family.

It is more of a dilemma for the professional when it is obvious that the parents have simply assumed that children should not attend funerals and have not considered the possible benefits of taking them. Should the parents' unconsidered judgement be challenged, or is this professional interference? The use of open questions is helpful here, for example:

'Have you thought about other options?'
'What has led you to make this decision?'

Professionals attending funerals

The public part of the funeral is the proper place for all affected by the death of the child to share their grief. Nurses, teachers, social workers, health visitors and doctors who have been closely involved with the child and family may wish to attend on their own behalf, or to represent their agency. Either way, it means a lot to the family to know that they were there. Rotas may limit the numbers of staff who can go, but managers who recognize the importance of key staff attending this ritual will try to accommodate their requests.

On first visiting the family

With or without previous knowledge of the family, the first visit to the home after the bereavement is fraught with anxiety. Typical concerns are:

- will the family welcome my visit?
- is it the right time to go?
- what can I say?
- will I be overwhelmed by their grief?

There is no magic formula to dispel the apprehension, but self-preparation can help to prevent unnecessary stress. Many of the following points relate to common sense and common good practice: but in the context of heightened emotions they can easily be forgotten.

Be realistic

Part of the anxiety comes from believing that you have to know the right thing to say that will help to ease their pain: so it is immediately freeing to acknowledge to yourself what an unrealistic expectation this is. Nothing you can say or do will help to bring back the life of the child, which would be the only thing to make the family 'feel better' at this time. You are guaranteed to feel helpless as a result.

Be realistic about the amount of follow-up support you can offer, so that you do not end up promising more than you can maintain.

Be prepared

It helps to double-check the information you have about the family, in particular the name and age of the child. Allow for more time than you might generally give to a home visit. If this is the first time you have been involved with the family, or when the death is sudden, it is likely that the full story needs to be told. To do justice to the child's memory and the parents' feelings, the story should not be rushed. Learning how to end your visit and when to withdraw is a skill that comes with experience! It is made easier if you say at the beginning what time is available to you. It is useful to remember that your visit will be emotionally draining for the family as well as for you. If you can, arrange your timetable so that you allow for the impact on you, by setting aside time afterwards to debrief with a colleague.

Be clear

Introduce yourself and say who you are representing. If you are not expected, check whether your visit at this time is convenient. The purpose of your visit may be obvious to you, but at a time of such confusion it is important to say what it is. In the first few days, the family may be visited by many different professionals and befrienders. It is helpful if you leave details of your name, organization, contact number and availability. Make it clear whether you will visit again, and if so, when that will be. An unscheduled visit from the GP or clergy can leave the family with unrealistic expectations of future visits which turn to disappointment. It is a good idea to follow up your first contact with a telephone call or a note if no other arrangement was made on your departure.

Be honest and genuine

The general principles detailed in Chapter 4 are all relevant, none more so than the warning against platitudes, which have a nasty habit of slipping out at times of anxiety. Nerves can also lead to inappropriate trading of your own experience, which should be firmly resisted, especially on this first visit. Bland reassurances do not comfort. A parent recalls the words of a visiting priest: 'You must remember that God's only son suffered on the cross for us.' The parent replied: 'Yes, but he didn't suffer for 18 months, like my son.'

If you feel lost for words, it does no harm to say so. A touch of the hand can say far more than words.

Accepting periods of silence and displays of emotion may be the most difficult but most valuable gift you can offer.

Anniversaries

Anniversaries are powerful replays of events and the emotions that accompanied them. Many parents find that the anticipation of the anniversary, during the preceding days, is as bad or worse than the day itself. Significant anniversaries also include the 'might-have-been' birthdays or other celebrations, as well as turning points in the terminal illness or events leading up to the death.

A contact of some kind by carers at the time of the anniversary of the death – particularly the first – is very much valued by the family, whether or not active support is ongoing. Many bereavement support organizations recommend a minimum of 13 months' support in order to help the bereaved through the first anniversary.

The contact that is made, by card, letter, telephone or visit, should always refer to the child by name. For example, the simplest wording on a card might be: 'To Andrew's family, with kind thoughts at this special time'.

If you are in regular contact with the family, do not be afraid of talking about the anniversary beforehand. Your support may be helpful in thinking through their options for marking the occasion, or in working out strategies for simply getting through the day.

For those who fantasize about rejoining their loved ones, the anniversary of the death may focus any suicidal thoughts. If your relationship with the parents allows, it is better to confront such thoughts than avoid them—see below.

Suicide risk assessment

Suicidal thoughts are common to bereaved parents, particularly in the first year of bereavement, and can be anticipated as normal. Contrary to public myth, you cannot put such ideas into people's heads by mentioning them. Fears of self-harm are generally diluted by talking about them and having them acknowledged. Although it is dangerous to generalize, the following pointers may help you to assess the risk of actual self-harm.

Usually a statement or implication of suicidal intent is concerned with ending one's misery than one's life. Typical comments are:

'I want to be with him and hold him again.'
'I want to go to bed and not wake up again.'
'Life is meaningless without him.'
'I can't go on like this.'
'He needs me more than the rest of the family.'

Such a remark needs an acknowledgement that you have heard the desperate feelings conveyed. An appropriate response might be:

'You sound as if you don't want to go on living – is that so?

If the reply is affirmative, the next step is to ask whether that means a conscious wish to die:

'Do you mean you want to end your life?'

This feels very risky, but be assured that in nearly all cases this question will draw a conditional response, such as:

'Yes, I think about it, but I wouldn't do anything because. . .'

Now you can relax, and safely invite further exploration of how those awful feelings are experienced, and try to convey some understanding of their validity. But what if your question draws a different response:

'Yes, I've thought it all out.' Or, simply, 'Yes.'

In this situation, the alarm bells are now ringing. Having gone so far, you need to follow with a question that will give a clear indication of purpose:

'Have you thought what you would do?'

Do not be afraid of asking this question, as it is key to the assessment of risk. The response may again be conditional:

'Well, I've thought of crashing the car, but I couldn't bear to hurt the rest of the family even more.'

Now you are dealing with some intent, balanced with reservations, which can be strengthened with your support. However, the response may be more specific:

> 'Oh yes. I have got the pills all saved up, and I know exactly how many to take.'

Such a detailed method needs to be taken as a serious statement of intent. This is rare, but if you are faced with this situation, *you must seek support and advice*. The ethical question of whether you should take any action without this person's consent needs to be considered. If you conclude that you should alert someone else with your worries, you must inform the person you are supporting that you are doing so out of concern for their safety and welfare.

Again, the need for good support and supervision for yourself is underlined by any doubts you may have on this score.

SECTION 3
Support for Families

6 Bereavement support strategies

The kind of support offered should ideally be determined by the needs of the bereaved, but realistically it will also depend on what resources are available. Different models for support services will be considered in the final chapter, but first it is necessary to describe the various approaches and what they aim to achieve. Other questions addressed are:

- how and when is this strategy appropriate?
- who offers this kind of help?
- how can this support be obtained?

Practical support

In the early days there is usually a need for practical support, particularly in the case of sudden death. Parents in extreme shock may find themselves unable to care adequately for their other children. They may find it hard to sleep, or to think about food, or to apply themselves to the practical arrangements that need to be made. The offer of a lift or childminding or the gift of a casserole can convey as much comfort as any words.

Ideally this kind of practical help is forthcoming from extended family, friends and neighbours who are sensitive to the parents' needs. However, not all parents want relief from practical tasks and would prefer to be busy doing things as a way of coping with the pain. It needs to be their choice. If in doubt, ask them. There is no virtue in guessing, although there is often an expectation that the professional should know what is best for other people.

Well-meaning relatives may be overzealous in their concern to protect their loved ones. An obvious example is the tendency for brothers and sisters of the dying or dead child being bundled away from the scene of action. Even at a very young age children will experience a sense of exclusion if they are 'sent away' at such a time. They may then feel somehow punished and guilty, but are likely to comply with the expectations of the adults around them that they should play nicely and not ask questions. Children learn quickly to protect their protectors. On the other hand, some children may be very relieved to have some respite from distress, and welcome the chance to stay with a favourite aunt for a break.

How does one know which course is preferred by a particular child? Ask the child. The experience of the Alder Centre staff was that even very young children, once freed of responsibility for 'looking after' their parents, know what they want and can be trusted to know what is right for them. If the possible alternatives are openly offered, for example 'Do you want to stay here with Mummy and Daddy tonight, or do you want to stay the night with Granny?', most children will give a truthful answer. As well as getting it right for the child, it is equally important to the child that she has been asked. The Centre's teenage siblings group also provided evidence of regrets which began, 'I wasn't even asked. . .'

An example of well-meaning relatives not taking account of a parent's wishes is given here by Joyce:

'I was 19 and unmarried when I had my first baby, and that was seen as a disgrace in those days. It was the year of the Aberfan tragedy. Catherine was born with the cord round her neck and she only lived 10 minutes. Somebody said: 'It's the best thing that could have happened'. There were complications so I had to stay in hospital for two weeks. My mum saw to the funeral and I only found out later where the baby was buried. The worst was when I got home: my mum had given everything away that I'd got ready for the baby – cot, pram, clothes, the lot. I know she thought she was doing it for the best, but I had nothing tangible left to connect with the baby and what I'd lost, nothing to grieve with.'

Not everyone has a good network of family support to fall back on. When this is the case, key community figures such as the clergy, church visitor or social worker will assume more significance in providing practical help.

Where several people are involved it is obviously important to co-ordinate efforts and to work co-operatively. As a primary health care manager, the family doctor might most naturally take on this co-ordinating role, although it could just as easily be the health visitor or social worker. The case for standardizing provision of care is argued at the end of the final chapter.

Whatever the role, any visitor to the home of a bereaved family is likely to feel apprehensive – may actually be terrified – about the level of distress within, and conscious of not knowing what to say or do to help. It takes courage to make the first call. However, having made contact, it is important only to offer support that can realistically be maintained.

Befriending

Several of the specialist support organizations, such as the Foundation for the Study of Infant Deaths, the Scottish Cot Death Trust, and The Compassionate Friends provide a valuable service. More generally The Samaritans may offer face-to-face contact as well as 24-hour crisis support by telephone. Hospices and church visitor schemes, and victim support organizations may also offer a befriending service.

Befriending is rather like a one-way friendship. The helper offers the acceptance and listening ear of a friend without the emotional ties which require mutuality. Talking has many therapeutic effects:

- it helps to accept the reality of the loss
- it is a way of expressing and discharging emotions
- it re-establishes order to a disorganized mind.

Most bereaved parents experience the need to go over and over the events surrounding the death and to talk about the baby or child in every detail. This can become wearing for relatives and friends. Not everyone is as fortunate as Rose:

'My sister and brother-in-law visited every evening from the day Paul was killed in September to Christmas. It was the highlight of my day, knowing that Betty was coming round and I could just be myself and talk about Paul.'

Jo and John faced a more usual situation:

'Our families and friends were very supportive at first, but after a few weeks, although people still asked how we were, nobody mentioned *David* any more, when we wanted to talk about him more than ever.'

Having permission and encouragement to talk are crucially important to all bereaved, and the more so when the bereavement is a social embarrassment. Providing that permission and encouragement are key tasks for befrienders. Their value should not be underestimated and this usually voluntary role can be difficult. It demands witnessing another's pain, being faced with unanswerable questions and being left with feelings of helplessness and inadequacy.

Preparation

Ideally the helper will have received some training in listening skills and at least some preparation for the implications of the role. The conditions of the befriending relationship need to be thought through beforehand regarding availability and expectations. Where does the contact take place? How long should one stay on a home visit? Is a home telephone number to be given out? The befriender will need support, and should not be left to ask for it if feeling under pressure. A built-in support system is the best way to ensure that the expectations of the role do not become overwhelming.

Who should take on this role?

As in other situations of adversity and trauma, one naturally turns to someone who has suffered a similar experience. There is a common bond which is conducive to trust and understanding. Therefore bereaved parents will often seek out contact with other parents to gain reassurance that they are not alone and that they can survive their tragedy.

If this support is being offered by bereaved parents, they obviously need to have reached the point where they can keep their own grieving separate when in this role. Nevertheless it is likely that their own grief will at times be re-awakened by another's pain, which again underlines the necessity for support.

Whether or not the befriender has lost a child, there is one golden rule: never to say, 'I know exactly how you feel.' This ranks as the cardinal sin of all platitudes. It robs the sufferer of the uniqueness of the individual experience.

When is befriending appropriate?

There is no proscribed time or circumstance, but the following could be taken as indicators.

- When the parent is not able to offload to family or friends.
- When the early support of family and friends has fallen off.
- When the parent is isolated or housebound.
- When the parent is struggling with the task of adjustment, practically or emotionally.
- When the parent is confronting difficult times such as an inquest, birthday, Christmas, anniversary.

Points to consider

- Is befriending appropriate?
- Is there a suitable helper available?
- Are the conditions of the relationship clear?
- Is there sufficient support for the befriender?

Counselling

Counselling has taken on a variety of meanings for different people, ranging from advice to long-term therapy. Basic assumptions are that counselling will provide *help* for someone with a *problem*, and that a trained counsellor will have the necessary *skills*. Referrals are often made by other professionals who feel out of their depth and lacking the competency required.

It seems important to examine these assumptions in an attempt to clarify the role of the bereavement counsellor and to arrive at some indicators as to when counselling is appropriate.

The purpose of counselling

In many contexts counselling is seen as a problem-solving activity, with the counsellor guiding the client towards resolution of the problem. This idea does not fit comfortably with bereavement, and yet the expectation of both client and referrer is often that the bereavement counsellor will do or say something to make things better. In fact, the focus of the work in all therapeutic counselling is with the client, who sets the pace and the agenda. A more useful view of bereavement counselling is that it provides a means of expressing grief and working on the tasks of mourning. For some, this may be the opportunity to deal with suppressed feelings of anger and despair. For others, bereavement will turn their world upside down in such a way that all areas of life are called into question – relationships, job, religion – and huge adjustments are required.

The loss of a child questions the meaning of life in a way that few would otherwise face. The loss of a child also contains a very special ingredient: that this child could have been the receiver and giver of the unconditional love we all crave. Thus the counselling relationship may be instrumental in rebuilding self-esteem and self-worth. The bereavement counsellor may become, for a while, the ideal parent we all wished we had and would like to be for our children.

The tasks of counselling

Grief counselling, then, may include any of the following tasks:

- coming to terms with the reality of the loss
- experiencing the pain of that loss
- adjusting to daily existence without the loved child
- making sense of a world that allowed such a tragic waste
- working out one's future direction and reason for living.

This was Barbara's experience:

'What brought me to counselling? I just seemed to be caught up in a dense fog which I could not escape from and at times this left me feeling totally lost and almost blind with panic. Counselling helped me to clear the fog and find the sky – even though the sky is still cloudy at times. Counselling has enabled me to sort through my jumbled experiences and feelings and recognize each for what it was. By recognizing these things I could deal with those that could be dealt with and learn to live with those that I cannot do anything about. Initially, it helped me to put some perspective into my life. I realized that I was not the only mother to have lost a baby. I directed my thoughts to one issue at a time and gradually I got some sense of control in my life. It has proved to be very liberating.'

The role of the counsellor

It follows from the above that the role of the bereavement counsellor is a demanding one and requires more than the use of counselling skills practised by many other helpers in the course of their work. This distinction is not a judgment of value, nor does it deny the competence of professionals who take on a counselling role without that 'specialist' job title. Indeed, there are many who by nature of their existing professional relationship with the bereaved, such as the GP, health visitor or social worker, are best placed to take it on. However, it is important to be clear about what the role requires and involves. It is misleading and irresponsible when people are described or describe themselves as bereavement counsellors on the basis of goodwill and a day's training in counselling skills. What, then, are the requirements for this role?

- Counsellors need to have done sufficient work on their own losses to be aware of their impact on their counselling.
- Counsellors need a level of training that has developed understanding of attachment and loss, the features of grief, the tasks of mourning and of the processes at work in the therapeutic relationship.
- Counsellors need a setting that gives clear boundaries to the work – a counselling 'contract' – particularly if they have other roles in relation to the client or patient.
- Counsellors need supervision to clarify the task in hand and to cope with the emotional demands and feelings of helplessness.

When is counselling appropriate?

As counselling is here defined as more in-depth than listening, more focused and detached than befriending, it follows that it is not appropriate in the early days of grief, not until the first traumatic shock-waves from the diagnosis or from the actual death have subsided. It would be like starting physiotherapy straight after breaking a leg, instead of allowing time for the initial healing to take place. It may be helpful to pursue this analogy, as not everyone needs physiotherapy after breaking a leg. With good health, good healing and good support one can learn to walk again unaided. However, if there are other injuries, if the healing is complicated, or if insufficient attention and time are given to the healing before weight-bearing, it is a different story. Similarly, the painful experience of losing a child may be complicated by particularly traumatic circumstances. It may re-awaken the pain of previous losses, losses that perhaps have not been acknowledged or resolved. Other demands of family or job may not allow time and opportunity to grieve, so that the painful feelings become suppressed. In these situations, the focused attention afforded by counselling can help to release the blockages to natural healing.

There are also special features associated with the loss of a child which may complicate grieving and may indicate a need of counselling. One such feature is the fear of insanity, which many parents experience. The frightening and unrelenting extremity of emotions, together with the inability to make sense of what has happened, can send the mind into chaos. Another common experience is feeling suicidal, sometimes driven by guilt, sometimes by a desire to be with the dead baby or child. These reactions are isolating and put a tremendous strain on relationships, between spouses, partners and with other family members. The counselling setting can provide a place of safety to discharge these tensions.

Availability of counselling

The first consideration is whether there is someone already involved and acceptable to the bereaved person who can meet the criteria given above, in terms of having awareness, training, time and supervision. If so, it is important that the counselling is set up separately from other activities, and has clear time limits. If these conditions are not met, it may be difficult for both to cope with the painful feelings aroused. Professionals for whom counselling is a secondary role will arrange to see someone at a time set aside for addressing the bereavement issues.

More and more health practices are employing trained counsellors, reflecting a more holistic approach to health and greater understanding of the relationship between emotional and physical well-being. In some parts of the UK there are bereavement centres or services with counsellors who have particular experience of working with grief. This was how Pam came to counselling:

> 'I lost my son 12 years ago. I thought I was managing OK but after a few years I was back and forth to the doctor's with one thing and another – pains across my shoulders, down my back, stomach-ache ... He was very good: in the end he said that either I went to a counsellor or he wouldn't be my GP any more! So I had no choice, though I didn't see it would do any good. In fact once I got there I realized how much I had been holding in and how much I needed

to talk about my feelings. I grieved in a way I hadn't allowed myself to do before. I still need to talk about Simon from time to time. If I don't, the feelings come from nowhere and hit me in the back of the neck.'

Where a referral system operates, it is important that the bereaved person is encouraged to self-refer, as it could be that a third party referral is more about the referrer's anxiety to help than the bereaved person's wish to be helped. Similarly, response to referrals should be directly with the bereaved, and thought given to how much information, if any, is shared with other professionals.

Where to refer?

Whatever the setting, how can the credibility and suitability of the counsellor be checked? Every counsellor, whether self-appointed or working within an organization, should be able to provide the enquirer with information about their code of ethics, training and ways of working.

Checklist of indicators for counselling

So many factors affect the course of grieving that it is impossible to predict who might benefit from counselling. However, here are some of the indicators:

- low self-esteem
- persistent suicidal feelings
- breakdown of relationships
- multiple or coincidental losses
- traumatic circumstances surrounding the death.

Psychotherapy

The distinction between counselling and therapy is a fine one. In the USA the words 'therapy' and 'therapist' are more or less synonymous with 'counselling' and 'counsellor' in the UK. To add to the confusion, some counsellors in the UK describe themselves as psychotherapists on the grounds that they are doing the same work.

What, then, is the difference? In terms of training, the psychotherapist is required to have undergone individual or group therapy and will have access to the psychodynamic approach, which facilitates the resolution of underlying conflicts of separation, probably from childhood. The psychotherapist is likely to work actively with the tranference of feelings that occur in the therapeutic relationship. Anyone with deep-seated personality problems would be better suited to this psycho-dynamic approach. The psychotherapist may use specialist techniques belonging to a particular school of therapy. The 'behavioural' approach, for example, may be useful to someone whose bereavement has led to entrenched phobic reactions, such as the panic attacks associated with agoraphobia.

At the same time, some trained counsellors will use the same assessment skills and range of techniques. This is a welcome reflection of the rising standards of professionalism in the counselling world. Unfortunately it leaves blurred edges between these two definitions and uncertainty about who to go to when more in-depth work is required. Reference to the British Association for Counselling Directory of Counsellors and Therapists may be helpful.

Psychology

Further distinctions need to be made for those seeking specialist help.

Generally speaking, referrals to a psychologist focus on behavioural concerns. Whilst the training for clinical psychology is traditionally behavioural in origin, the psychologist is not restricted to this approach. Referrals are assessed individually and the appropriate therapy is offered. Where children are concerned, this may take the form of play therapy, or work with the whole family. Referral to a clinical psychologist can be made through the GP or, in some cases, directly to the psychology service at the hospital.

When the help of a child psychologist is engaged for grieving siblings who show distressing and persistent behavioural changes, it is essential that such help is seen by the child as supportive. Otherwise there is the real danger that the child is scapegoated for the parents' or family's difficulties and will be labelled as a 'problem'.

Psychiatry

Traditional psychiatric support is seen to be appropriate in the context of mental illness, and concentrates on drug treatments. Although many bereaved parents do, for a time, experience mental chaos and fear they are going mad, this is different from the long-term separation from reality that accompanies psychotic illness. Also, the depression which normally accompanies bereavement – the suppressing of painful feelings – needs to be distinguished from depressive illness, which is physically dysfunctional and requires medical treatment.

However, in some hospitals and child guidance centres, psychiatrists who work alongside psychologists and social workers offer a more flexible response and make use of other therapeutic skills. This multi-disciplinary approach is also commonly used for family therapy. This may be the desired option when the death of a child results in family dysfunction. It has obvious advantages when one member of the family – usually another child – is carrying responsibility for all the family's distress. The desired outcome of involving all or some of the family members is to help each one acknowledge feelings and be acknowledged – thus helping the family adjust to its loss. Family therapy may be available through the local health services, social services and voluntary agencies such as Barnardo's and the Children's Society.

Finally, a word about the value of these different therapeutic approaches. It is hard to get away from the assumption that those practitioners who have had more specialized training and are better paid also offer 'better' services. The worth of any counselling or therapy depends on the quality of the attention given to the bereaved person or family.

The word therapist comes from the ancient Greek 'therapon', a servant who freely chose to devote his life to giving attention to others' needs. To make the same point in another way, as the antipsychiatrist RD Laing said 'Treatment is about how you treat people'. The core qualities of warmth, empathy and respect form the basis of any supportive relationship. Carol found these qualities in her befriender:

> 'Jenny saw me through the worst time, really. For the first months after James died I couldn't go out, not even to the shops. I felt I couldn't face anyone. I rang the Alder Centre helpline one evening, and after that Jenny came to see me every week till I got my confidence back. She knew just what I was going through, because she'd been there too. And I remember thinking, she's survived, so maybe I will.'

Groups

Meeting together with others to form a group is a powerful experience. This is particularly true for those who feel isolated by the shattering effects of losing a child. Common bonds are formed by that shared experience which cut across differences in age, social status, education and religion. It can be enormously reassuring and enabling to hear others express similar thoughts and feelings, and to know they face similar difficulties. It can provide a safe environment for dropping the public mask of normality and owning inner struggles with pain, anger, guilt and frustration. Negatives are balanced by positives, so that one member can feed off another's hope or optimism.

Lin's daughter Yvonne, aged 15, was killed in a road accident while on holiday abroad. She turned to the Alder Centre for support, and these are her recollections about attending the Open House group:

'It saved my sanity. I felt very lonely, and I used to feel as if I was going mad, talking to Yvonne as if she was still in the house; but when I heard others say similar things, I thought "Thank God, it happens to them too". I felt I could just be *me* there, whether in a happy mood or at rock bottom. I could laugh without feeling apologetic, and cry without feeling ashamed.'

Groups can also be extremely threatening for the same reason, that shared feelings are intensified. For some, particularly in the early days of bereavement, it is just too much to consider anyone else's pain but one's own. Timing and preparation are therefore important for anyone joining a group. The nature of the group will also affect the outcome. Does it have a therapeutic purpose, or is it focused on shared activities? Is it exclusive to parents, to adults, or to families? Are affected children to be offered a separate group? Alder Centre staff, acutely aware of the often overlooked needs of siblings, formed a discussion group for bereaved teenagers, which proved shortlived (eight months) and limited in its usefulness. This experience pointed towards activity as a more suitable focus for this age group, as described on page 111.

Self-help groups

The main focus of the self-help group is mutual support. The structure is usually informal and the agenda set by the members. It often provides a network of support outside the group meetings, leading to new friendships. Although there is freedom from the leadership of outside helpers, someone will need to take on a facilitator role in terms of liaison and organization. One model for self-help groups for bereaved parents is provided by The Compassionate Friends, with local co-ordinators who act as contact points.

One advantage of self-selection is the potential for minority groups to meet together. At the Alder Centre three mothers were introduced to each other who had lost a teenage son through suicide. They decided to meet regularly to support each other over a period of months and gained great comfort from this. At another time a similar minigroup formed itself comprised of parents of murdered children.

Led groups

Support groups set up by professional or voluntary workers offer the security of leadership, which helps to facilitate the work of the group. The formation of the group may be in response to request or perceived need. The role of the leader(s) may be a passive one, keeping time boundaries and facilitating introductions; or it may be more directive, with structured meetings around themes or tasks. In any case the leader will act as a kind of container for the group which makes it a very stressful role. The importance of planning, clear aims, ground rules and good support/supervision for the leaders cannot be overestimated, and these issues will be addressed in the next chapter. Obviously a therapeutic group requires skilled leadership.

The advantage of led groups for the members is that they are released from responsibility for the group and feel safer to express difficult feelings. There will also be a degree of detachment in the leader, which enables them to orchestrate the group, so that everyone who wishes to speak has an opportunity to be heard.

Structure – open or closed?

An open group is one that has a fluctuating membership, open to all-comers with a free option whether and when to attend. This flexibility is welcome to those who feel the need for support at particular times, and may not wish to attend when they are feeling specially vulnerable or when they are enjoying a 'good patch'. If there is no consistent core of members, however, it can be difficult for newcomers to build trust in the group. The fact that newcomers are joining the group all the time also means that open groups go on from week to week or month to month, without any natural end. Newer members may welcome this, reassured by the presence of bereaved people who are further on in their journey: longer-term members may eventually find it less helpful to be constantly drawn back to the early days of grieving. On the other hand, an open group has the advantage of doing away with expectations about how anyone should be or behave according to the length of their bereavement.

A closed group is one that has a selected membership over a fixed period of time, and is likely to be more structured than an open group. A fixed term group is the preferred choice of most professionals who act as facilitators for several reasons:

- it is more manageable in terms of their own commitment
- it promotes trust and continuity for the members, who are therefore able to risk more of their true feelings
- it prevents dependence
- it confronts the harsh reality of moving on.

A closed group seems more appropriate for those who share common features in their bereavement, for example a group of parents who have lost a child from the same illness in the same hospital over the same period of time. It is perhaps less appropriate for those whose loss leaves little chance of adjustment, such as parents who have lost an older child for whom they have cared over many years.

It is worth recording that after three years' experience of a whole range of different closed and open groups, the Alder Centre staff became convinced of the advantages of setting limits on the life of a group, whether that marks the end of the group or provides a natural break before reconvening.

Social activities

Shared activity can be a wonderful therapy in its own right. It is particularly attractive to those who have no time for counselling or groups but who welcome the chance to mix with others who share their special experience. Social events, physical activity, fund-raising organization and committee work all provide the opportunity for oblique support. Purposeful activity seems to be a natural coping mechanism for many men who are distrustful of emotion or see themselves in the stronger supportive role in the family.

Children are usually better disposed towards doing things than talking about feelings they are unsure about. A year after the Alder Centre teenagers group folded, two expeditions to Northumberland to swim with Freddie the dolphin proved enormously popular and provided the opportunity for bereaved siblings to share experiences that had marked them out in another way. Planning and preparation brought them together socially, and the encounters with Freddie gave them a sense of being special as well as different. For one of those youngsters, the adventure also gave her the confidence to talk about the death of her sister for the first time. Their families came together to watch video recordings and share photographs. Virginia McKenna visited the Centre to talk to a couple of these dolphin-swimmers as research for her book . . . and so the spin-offs continued.

As well as reducing isolation, social activities for adults can be fun too! Quiz nights, country walks and shared holidays bring people together to enjoy the good things of life. These are not only welcome diversions but also affirmations of one's place in the world and the right to take pleasure in it alongside the pain of grief. This was the comment of one mother after a week spent in the Lake District with other parents:

'I now know the meaning of holidays and what they are for, which since the death of my child I had forgotten.'

The Alder Centre has also organized shared family holidays, providing encouragement as well as opportunity to enjoy again an activity which may have lost its meaning.

Support for children

Various references have been made to the difficulties surrounding children's support needs. Parents who are overwhelmed by their own grief may find it hard to attend to the needs of their surviving children. Adults struggle to gain access to the understanding and feelings of children who have not developed the emotional language to express themselves. Children seek to protect their carers from distress as much as their carers try to shield them from the painful reality of death. As a result, children often become 'the forgotten mourners' when a sibling or friend dies. For those helpers who are aware of children's needs, the question remains of how to provide for them – particularly when dealing with very young children – which will avoid problems later on.

The most important factor which determines how children cope with loss is the attitude of the parents. Young children suffer most the *secondary* losses, such as lack of attention and the loss of security in an ordered world, when a sibling dies. If the parents are able to include their other children in their experience of loss, keeping them involved and informed, while at the same time maintaining a sense of safety and security in the family, then they will cope well. Parents are best placed to answer a child's questions and provide reassurance to counter their fears and concerns.

It follows, then, that the best way of supporting children is through the parents. First of all that means providing adequate support for the parents. Most of the anxious parents who brought young children to the Alder Centre for help were unwittingly asking for help for themselves. The attention given to one mother who had not had time to grieve for her baby stopped her seven-year-old son's bedwetting. The space given to one couple to air their marital tensions after losing a child dissipated the aggressive behaviour of their five-year-old daughter.

Second, parents can be briefed as to how best to support their other children at the time of the bereavement. Remind parents that children will 'read' the emotions around them and overhear conversations, and will ask questions either directly or indirectly. The Foundation for the Study of Infant Deaths and cot death associations have highlighted the needs of siblings, publishing leaflets and training befrienders to raise the issues with parents. The Compassionate Friends also publish helpful articles on the grief of sibling children and teenagers and how to help them to understand death.

Advice to parents for the benefit of children

- If at all possible, keep the family together.
- Keep children informed about what is happening. Even very young children will sense distress and need to know its cause. It is better

for children to hear unpleasant things from their parents than from strangers.

- Answer children's questions as honestly as you can.
- Reassure them that the death of their brother or sister was not their fault or responsibility.
- Do not be afraid of using the word 'death'. Children get confused and worried by phrases like 'gone to sleep' or 'taken by Jesus'. Avoid fairy tales to explain death, and do not be afraid to admit that you do not know all the answers. The more openly your family can talk about death, the easier it is for the child to accept it.
- Allow your children to feel sad, angry and all the natural feelings of grief, although do not expect them to feel sad all the time.
- When young children include some aspect of the death in their play, this is normal and healthy. The same goes for telling strangers 'My little brother is dead'.
- Do not be afraid to show your own grief in front of your children. This will help them to grieve, and reassure them that you loved the child who died.
- Give constant reassurance that you love and care equally for these children too. Give them special times, and listen.
- Do ask for help if you feel unable to deal with your children during this time.

If parents are not able to be the primary carers for a while, or are emotionally incapable of giving this kind of attention, then many of the above tasks can be undertaken by a relative. The family may enrol the help of a member of the clergy, a teacher, a social worker or a health visitor to talk to a child or answer her questions. This should always be done in consultation with the parents, and if possible in their presence.

How far should a professional take the initiative in cases where the parents seem unaware of their child's needs? Such situations require great sensitivity in explaining to parents the cause for concern and gaining their co-operation. Working with the parents to win their trust brings the best chance of success.

In any case, talking to a child about death and allowing the expression of bereft feelings cannot be done in a vacuum. It needs to be done within the context of a trusting and caring relationship, with time for the child to talk and react.

Explaining death to children

Children's concepts of death vary according to age and experience. They are often distorted, but are usually more developed than adults appreciate (*see* Chapter 2, pages 38–40).

The most common emotions for children are fear and anxiety, as fertile imaginations grapple with the unknown. As adults, we are not immune from these anxieties, which inhibit our ability to answer children's questions. Dogmatic beliefs about immortality are not helpful to children who are as yet unable to think in abstract terms, nor are they likely to be reassured by the bald statement 'I don't know'. Offering ideas to children, which are drawn from their own experience, and asking for *their* ideas leads to helpful exploration.

The most common confusion is about death and sleep, and the difference between them needs to be clearly explained. It may help to say that the body stops working when a person dies, so that he does not need to sleep any more.

Most children want to know what happens to dead people. Whatever ideas are used here, it is reassuring to children to distinguish somehow between the body, which decays or is burned, and the spirit of a person, which continues. An analogy that is often used is the difference between a house and a home, although children create the best images themselves to express this idea.

The best explanations are simple, unambiguous, and drawn from the child's own experience. Bearing in mind the capacity of young children to have 'magical thoughts', it is important to check that what you have told the child is what she has actually heard, to avoid misunderstandings.

Behavioural reactions

The range of emotions and anxieties that children experience may be reflected in various behaviours. It is reassuring to parents and professionals alike to know that any of the following reactions are common:

- anxiety about being separated from parents
- difficulty in going to sleep
- fear of the dark
- regressing to an earlier stage, such as clinging or talking in a baby voice, or wetting the bed
- a tendency to infections
- reluctance to go to school
- difficulty in concentrating
- overeating, or a loss of interest in food
- developing a phobia about doctors or hospitals
- angry outbursts
- withdrawal
- depression.

It is not so much the presence of these behaviours but their persistence over a long period that makes them a cause for concern, when they indicate a need for specialist support.

Cultural differences

All the support strategies described in this chapter are designed to reduce the isolation of those who are bereaved by the death of a child. For those who already belong to a minority group, the isolation will be intensified and they will find it harder to tap into the available resources. In multicultural Britain, most resources are geared towards white, middle-class, conventional families. To declare one's grief is also to display one's differences. If those differences outweigh the shared experience of losing a child, each culture will have to provide its own resources until a better day dawns on integration.

Certainly, each culture has much to learn from others. The Alder Centre outreach work in local communities and independent research projects attempted to explore the reasons why so few black parents made contact. Several requests for help from Muslim women could not be followed up for fear of their family's disapproval. The single visit of an Asian woman was particularly distressing. She had returned to the hospital to visit the ward where her son died and collect his belongings, and called at the Centre in floods of tears. She wanted to see the Book of Remembrance. When follow-up support was offered, she declined: she had to keep this visit a secret for fear of being punished by her husband for seeking help outside the family. Undoubtedly the Alder Centre has not been accessible to many black families because it does not present a multicultural image. At the same time, white Europeans have much to learn from other ethnic groups about the spontaneous expression of grief and the strength of family support.

Further reading

Green J (1991) Death with dignity: meeting the spiritual needs of patients in a multi-cultural society. *Nursing Times*.

Grollman EA (1990) *Talking about death: a dialogue between parent and child*. Beacon Press, Boston.

Neuberger J (1987) *Caring for dying people of different faiths*. Austen Cornish, London.

Speck P (1978) *Loss and grief in medicine*. Bailliere Tindall, London.

7   Guidelines for support services

As the special needs of bereaved families become better recognized, various initiatives are developed to provide support. Some thrive while others prove short-lived, and the difference between the two is often put down to chance. It will be proposed here that the success of any support service will depend first on meeting certain core conditions, and second on good planning and preparation. These will be applied to the setting up of a support group, but could equally well be applied to starting a helpline or befriending service.

The Alder Centre in Liverpool has been used as a model for similar projects offering co-ordinated services to those affected by the death of a child, and the Preface to this book records its development. The valuable lessons that have been learned are offered in the hope of encouraging other multidisciplinary approaches involving parent participation. Finally, the way forward to improve bereavement care will focus on the need for co-ordinated services, better information and pro-active support.

Core conditions

Some basic principles apply to the establishment of any support service, whether it be a group, befriending, counselling or a multipurpose centre.

Identifying the need

This means consulting those who are perceived as needing support at the time. One difficulty is that people do not always know what they want in their distress, or whether the support being offered will suit them. In this case the helper can draw on past experience of families and consult other professionals. Another possible factor is that well meaning carers may be more concerned about 'doing something to help' than responding to actual need. Indeed, an assessment of support needs may indicate a separate agenda for the professional or volunteer, which will have to be recognized and accommodated. Assessment also involves identifying existing means of support, to ensure that services are not duplicated.

Sufficiency of resources

Too often, bereavement support initiatives fizzle out for want of adequate resources. Perhaps after a first flush of enthusiasm, just a few volunteers are left to cope with too many demands. Sometimes an initiative will depend on the commitment of one dedicated individual, whose bereavement work is not recognized as part of the job: when that person moves on, the project collapses. Sufficiency of resources relates to people, time, space and money. Although the setting up of any new service requires an act of faith, it is irresponsible to do so without reasonable confidence that the service can be sustained over a period of time, especially when working with loss and grief.

Support systems

Care for the carers is essential in such an emotionally demanding area of work. Management and administrative structures are necessary to any support system, however informal.

Key questions need to be addressed at the research and planning stage relating to the type and scope of the proposed service.

- At whom is the service aimed?
- What does the service aim to achieve?
- What are the geographical boundaries?
- What is already being done?
- What is the preferred setting?
- Who will deliver the service?
- What are the criteria for taking referrals?
- Who will manage and supervise the work?

At all stages it is important to work co-operatively with those with common interests and seek their support. Bereavement projects, by nature of the subject, tend to attract defensive attitudes! Canvassing for a broad base of support also ensures that your plans are in line with progressive thinking and good practice in other areas.

Starting a support group

The guidelines suggested here assume that professional or voluntary workers are responding to perceived needs of bereaved family members, which may be met by offering a group experience. For the sake of convenience I shall refer to the potential group participants as parents, although of course they may be grandparents or siblings. The process will be the same, except that a sibling group will need parental agreement, and its leaders will require some understanding of children's perceptions.

Identifying the need

The impetus to start a group tends to fall into one of three categories.

1. In response to requests from parents to meet other parents for mutual support.
2. In anticipation of griefwork which can be facilitated in a therapeutic setting.
3. As an economical way of coping with limited resources to offer individual help.

Being clear about the purpose will affect the direction you take and determine the appropriate type of group (*see* Chapter 6 for an outline of different group types). Whatever the impetus, it is important not to be pressured into starting a group before adequate preparation. This may be frustrating for potential participants, who will welcome regular communication during the planning stages.

The consultation process includes an audit of what is happening elsewhere to avoid duplicating resources, and making links with other colleagues, agencies and disciplines to ensure a broad base of support for the venture. Management may require data to back up any application for time or other resources and to clarify issues such as confidentiality.

Calling a meeting

An open meeting of all interested parties needs a clear agenda, someone to take a chairing role and someone to take names and notes. If likely attenders of the group are not present, their views should be represented.

The primary purpose of this first meeting is to take an audit of concerns, current practice, interests and resources.

- It is helpful to begin with introductions by name, role, agency representation and reason for attending. Some may see this initiative as a means of getting recognition of the work they already do for bereaved families or to gain understanding of their own support needs: it is important that these concerns are acknowledged by the Chair so that they can be openly identified and separated from the parents' needs.
- The purpose of the group, in the kind of general terms that can be summarized in one sentence, should then be agreed.

- The type and status of group required can then be discussed, along with the implications for resources. It may not be possible to reach a consensus at this stage.
- Another audit follows of the kind of help and commitment attenders are willing and able to give.
- A *small* working party can now take the findings forward to the next planning stage. There tends to be a high level of enthusiasm at this first meeting, so beware the 'hands up to volunteer' approach! Some means of communicating progress needs to be agreed, and dates set if the working party is to report back to another general meeting.

Planning

The planning tasks cover objectives, method, structure and programme, and a number of meetings may be needed.

- *Objectives:* these spell out the aim and purpose in specific terms. What will the group need to achieve its purpose? What conditions need to be met?
- *Method:* what kind of group (open or closed, self-help or led, spontaneous or planned) will be most appropriate? What size, composition and setting will help to meet the objectives?
- *Structure:* this provides boundaries for the group and moves on to practicalities. These will include:
  - setting dates for starting (and finishing)
  - deciding the venue
  - agreeing the personnel to facilitate the group
  - guidelines for access, referral and selection
  - publicity
  - arranging support and supervision for leaders
  - setting dates for evaluation.
- *Programme:* the facilitators/leaders of the group will need to be involved, if not already part of the working party, to plan timing, format and – if appropriate – the content of group meetings. If canvassing for participants, a rough guide to uptake is that one in three will respond. Parents who wish to attend the group should be visited beforehand if possible.

Delivery

Thought needs to be given to the preparation of the room, who will welcome the group members, how the group will start and how it will end. Finishing group meetings can be very difficult, but it is important to draw the session to a close, gently but firmly, at the time stated. Groups that go on till midnight are exhausting for all concerned. Parents who are overwhelmed by exposure to never-ending pain are likely to drop out. It helps if the facilitator signals the end of the session some minutes beforehand, and at the finish time physically leaves the room or puts the kettle on.

It is essential for those in charge of the meeting, whether called hosts, leaders or facilitators, to debrief their feelings and reactions before going home and ensure that time for this is built in.

Evaluation

Groups do not always turn out as expected, even after meticulous planning! Evaluation is part of the group process, and may lead to amendments as the group goes on. At another level, the facilitators' supervisor will help them to evaluate their contribution, celebrating achievements as well as learning from mistakes. Managers and funding bodies may also require evaluative reports. When the group is time-limited, evaluation may lead to the implementation of necessary changes if another group is proposed. Open-ended groups benefit from a break of some kind, perhaps over the summer, which provides a natural time for taking stock.

A co-ordinated approach

Lessons and recommendations from the Alder Centre experience

The success story of the Alder Centre has depended on a great deal of good will and generosity. Operating a true partnership of parents and professionals is very hard work for all concerned, but offers a way of working which embodies respect, empathy and genuineness, and is very rewarding.

Partnership

Parents have guided the development of the Centre's policy and practice to make the services relevant to their needs. Professionals offer detachment, particular skills and expertise, but are always accountable to their 'clients' in a direct way. The principle of partnership demands a consultative and consensual style of management.

Parent participation has proved therapeutic, whether as conference speaker or tea-maker. Helping others gives more purpose and meaning to the lives they are rebuilding.

Dot is one of the parents who has worked tirelessly for the centre since the planning stage. As her 13-year-old daughter was approaching death, Dot asked her, 'What do you want me to do?' Christine's answer was, 'Help someone else.' In the volunteer tasks Dot has undertaken – answering the telephone, befriending, fund raising, talking to visitors and co-ordinating publicity – she feels that her child has been working alongside her. This feeling is shared by many of the parent volunteers.

Place

Having a geographical base with salaried staff ensures continuity. The Centre provides far more than a model of mental health care: its very existence challenges taboos about child death and legitimizes the concerns of bereaved families. It affirms the good work being done by individuals and groups in the wider community, and promotes the training and support needs of professionals.

Planning

The benefits of thorough preparation showed up in the following ways.

- A broad base of support across all disciplines and parts of the community ensured co-operation and maximized resources.
- A clear remit provided safe boundaries within which to work.
- The appointment of non-medical staff freed parents to vent anger and freed staff from involvement in medical or legal issues.
- The appointment of staff who were not bereaved parents themselves freed parents of anxiety about staff reactions.
- Built-in provision of an independent supervisor for the counselling staff proved essential to their well-being.

Difficulties

Progress was not always smooth. As with any 'family' concern, tensions are bound to arise. The structure of the enterprise threw up issues which had to be worked through.

Ownership

The initial lack of a constitution for the Advisory Group and contract with the hospital authorities created uncertainty about autonomy and decision-making.

Management

The dual role of manager and counsellor demanded a wide range of different skills and qualities to maintain the Centre's egalitarian approach within a clear structure.

Responsibility

Dilemmas arose about the Centre's level of responsibility for Centre activities not facilitated by the staff, and for affiliated community groups. Copyright of logo and training materials had to be considered.

Priorities

The flexibility to run a drop-in centre that also guaranteed appointment times often proved stressful. Referral systems and assessment procedures ensured a measured response, with built-in flexibility to respond immediately to those in acute distress, but unpredictable situations could stretch staff and volunteers to the limit. As the training function grew, there was a tension between the aims of providing support and raising awareness.

Protection
Staff endeavoured not to take on a parental role towards volunteers, but at times felt bound to protect parents from exploitative media exposure.

Integration
Founder parents had a vested interest in continuing links with the Centre as a place of their own, while many newcomers tended to move away once they felt they had received the support they wanted at critical times. Integrating old and new parents posed challenges as their needs diverged.

What other lessons have been learned?

Every service creates another level of need
Professionals who help to run groups and volunteers who do befriending will need support for themselves. Volunteer training opens the door to self-awareness and further training needs. Those referring another for help usually have needs of their own, and the staff learned to take this into account when responding to third party referrals.

Good quality equipment and materials reinforce people's worth
It is tempting to cut corners where voluntary funding is concerned, but you really do get what you pay for. Good salaries attract good staff; good quality stationery, publications and training materials gain credibility; and above all, a comfortable environment tells visitors they are valued and respected.

Staff training and support needs are crucially important
The first staff change resulted in redefining the outreach post as an outreach counsellor, in recognition of the need for counselling training for all direct work undertaken by staff. This kind of work demands a high degree of self-awareness and the ability to separate oneself from others' pain.

Efficient systems put people first
Clear procedures, guidelines and good record-keeping allow carers to be spontaneous and creative within safe limits.

Client-centred helping approaches really work
This means respecting everyone's uniqueness and self-direction, and believing in their ability to know what is right for them. The Centre counsellors learned not to underestimate their capacity to help by giving people that respect and faith.

The way forward

How can support services for those affected by the death of a child be improved? At present the support available to a bereaved family, and to their carers, seems to be a random affair, depending on where people live. Comprehensive systems like the Alder Centre are probably only practicable in association with a children's hospital or hospice. Those living in a sparsely populated rural area have a slim chance of finding a support group within easy travelling distance. On the other hand, everyone has access to primary health care services and, through them, should have access to regional and national services. It is hoped that this book will give confidence to professionals to co-ordinate and advertise existing resources, and to experiment with more pro-active means of support.

The need for co-ordinated services

In the experience of the Alder Centre, whenever a new support group was initiated on Merseyside, other individuals and groups identified themselves as offering support to bereaved families, often working in isolation. Telephone enquirers from other parts of the country were often surprised to hear of professional and voluntary services located in their area, which were known to the Centre.

There is a clear case to be made for some means of auditing and co-ordinating bereavement support services at a regional level, to work towards a standard provision of care. This could start with an agreed protocol for hospitals in the event of a child's death, leading on to procedures for liaison with community services and ongoing care providers. Regional health authorities are best placed to take this on, but funding for regional co-ordinator posts would need to be found.

The need for better information

'If only I had known . . .' is a common refrain from bereaved parents. Again, it seems to be the luck of the draw whether the child's hospital staff, the family's GP or the health visitor have access to the information that the family can use. Primary health care workers need to be as well informed about bereavement care services as about the side-effects of drugs. There is an equal obligation on such services to make themselves known and familiar, not only to health centres but also to the Citizen's Advice Bureau, Samaritans, libraries and the local media.

Pro-active support

The usual expectation of the agency is that bereaved parents themselves make contact, or that a third party referral is received by a concerned professional, friend or relative. Yet it is well known that the bereavement experience leaves many parents paralysed by shock, floating in a limbo of grief that renders them incapable of asking for help. Agoraphobic responses to grief are common. Members of minority groups are naturally reluctant to use mainstream services. All these factors beg the question of whether support services should initiate contact – or whether this would amount to an invasion of privacy.

The Kinder–Mourn Project in North Carolina, USA, is a community support agency modelled on The Compassionate Friends, but uses facilitators who will *initiate* contact with bereaved parents brought to their attention by anyone concerned for their welfare. Home visits as early as the day of the funeral point the way towards informal parent support groups led by trained facilitators. Leaving aside the fact that parents are charged fees on a sliding scale for this service, the Kinder–Mourn approach has much to recommend it.

In our naturally conservative British society, outreach is an unfamiliar concept; but arguably there is much to be achieved by support agencies reaching out to those who are unable to ask for help themselves.

The guidelines offered here aim to encourage the faint-hearted as well as the visionary, and to affirm the good practice of those already engaged in providing bereavement services. These observations will allow readers to make a realistic assessment of possible means of support that they can provide themselves, and give an overview of support strategies available from other sources.

Support is a two-way process. Families want information, choices and understanding. Professional carers need assurance that they *can* and *do* help by providing that information and choice, and above all by being available to accompany the family on their journey through grief.

Further reading

Stewart J (1991) *Guidelines for setting up a bereavement counselling or support service*. National Association of Bereavement Services, London.

Further Reading

Bluebond-Langner M (1978) *The private worlds of dying children.* Princeton University Press, Princeton.

Bowlby J (1991) *Attachment and loss*, vol 1, 2nd edn. Penguin, Harmondsworth.

Cook B and Phillips S (1988) *Loss and bereavement.* Austen Cornish, London.

Donnelly KF (1988) *Recovering from the loss of a sibling.* Dodd Mead, New York.

Green J (1991) Death with dignity: meeting the spiritual needs of patients in a multi-cultural society. *Nursing Times.*

Grollman EA (1990) *Talking about death.* Beacon, Boston.

Gullo S (1985) *Death and children.* Dobbs Ferry, New York.

Jewett C (1984) *Helping children cope with separation and loss.* Batsford, London.

Knight B (1983) *Sudden death in infancy.* Faber & Faber, London.

Kohner N and Henley A (1991) *When a baby dies.* Stillbirth and Neonatal Death Society, London.

Kubler-Ross E (1970) *On death and dying.* Tavistock Press, London.

Lendrum S and Syme G (1992) *Gift of tears.* Routledge, London.

Littlewood J (1992) *Aspects of grief.* Routledge, London.

McCollum A (1975) *The chronically ill child: a guide for parents and professionals.* Yale University Press, New Haven.

Neuberger J (1987) *Caring for dying people of different faiths.* Austen Cornish, London.

Oakley A *et al.* (1984) *Miscarriage.* Fontana, London.

Parkes CM (1972) *Bereavement.* Pelican, Harmondsworth.

Pincus L (1976) *Death and the family.* Faber & Faber, London.

Raphael B (1984) *The anatomy of bereavement: a handbook for the caring professions.* Unwin Hyman, London.

Sanders P (1993) *A complete guide to using counselling skills on the telephone.* PCCS Books, Manchester.

Shawe M (Ed.) (1992) *Enduring, sharing, loving.* Darton, Longman & Todd, London.

Speck P (1978) *Loss and grief in medicine.* Bailliere Tindall, London.

Stedeford A (1984) *Facing death: patients, families and professionals.* Heinemann, Oxford.

Stewart J (1991) *Guidelines for setting up a bereavement service.* National Association of Bereavement Services, London.

Tatelbaum J (1981) *The courage to grieve.* Heinemann, Oxford.

Vachon M (1981) *Occupational stress in the care of the critically ill, the dying and the bereaved.* Hemisphere, Washington DC.

Ward B *et al.* (1992) *Good grief: exploring feelings, loss and death (i. over elevens and adults, ii. under elevens)*, 2nd edn. Jessica Kingsley, London.

Worden JW (1991) *Grief counselling and grief therapy*, 2nd edn. Routledge, London.

Useful addresses

The organizations listed below are either mentioned in the text or have a principal concern to support bereaved families and/or health and care professionals.

ACT (Association for Children with Terminal and life-threatening conditions and their families) – umbrella organization providing information about available services.
Institute of Child Health, Royal Hospital for Sick Children,
St Michael's Hill, Bristol BS2 8BJ.
Tel: (0272) 221556.

Alder Centre – for *all* those affected by the death of a child, providing support, information and training.
Royal Liverpool Children's NHS Trust, Alder Hey, Eaton Road,
Liverpool L12 2AP.
Tel: (051) 252 5391.

Alder Centre Helpline   7–10 p.m. every evening.
Tel: (051) 228 9759.

Association for Children with Heart Disorders – support for families with children suffering heart disorders.
26 Elizabeth Drive, Helmshaw, Rossendale, Lancashire BB4 4JB.
Tel: (0706) 213 632.

British Association for Counselling
1 Regent Place, Rugby CV21 2PJ.
Tel: (0788) 578328.

Cancer Relief Macmillan Fund – funds Macmillan nurses to give advice and support for cancer patients and their families.
Anchor House, 15/19 Britten Street, London SW3 3TZ.
Tel: (071) 351 7811.

Compassionate Friends (TCF) – nationwide self-help organization for bereaved parents; resource library and advice leaflets.
53 North Street, Bristol BS3 1EN.
Tel: (0272) 539639.

Cystic Fibrosis Trust – research, support and education.
Alexandra House, 5 Blyth Road, Bromley, Kent BR1 3RS.
Tel: (081) 464 7211.

Foundation for the Study of Infant Deaths – research, support, information and good practice guidelines.
5 Belgrave Square, London SW1X 8QB.
Tel: (071) 235 0965.

Great Ormond Street Helpline   7–10 p.m. Mondays and Thursdays.
Tel: (071) 829 8685.

ISIDA   (Irish Sudden Infant Death Association)
Carmichael House, 4 North Brunswick Street, Dublin 7.
Tel: (outside Ireland) (010) 3531 732711.

Laura Centre – for *anyone* affected by the death of a child, providing support and supervision.
4 Tower Street, Leicester LE1 6WS.
Tel: (0533) 544341.

Malcolm Sargent Cancer Fund for Children – assisting all young people under 21 with any form of cancer and their families.
14 Abingdon Road, London W8 6AF.
Tel: (071) 937 4548.

Miscarriage Association
c/o Clayton Hospital, Northgate, Wakefield, West Yorkshire WF1 3JS.
Tel: (0924) 200799.

NABS   (National Association of Bereavement Services) – referral agency and training information.
20 Norton Folgate, Bishopsgate, London E1 6DB.
Tel: (071) 247 0617.

NASS   (National Association for Staff Support within the health care services).
9 Caradon Close, Woking, Surrey GU21 3DU.
Tel: (0483) 771599.

SANDS   (Stillbirth And Neonatal Death Society) – support, information and guidelines.
28 Portland Place, London W1N 4DE.
Tel: (071) 436 7940.

SANDS Helpline Tel: (071) 436 5881.

SATFA (Support After Termination For Abnormality) – individual and group support for parents.
29–30 Soho Square, London W1V 6JB.
Tel: (071) 439 6124 (Parents)
Tel: (071) 287 3753 (Admin)

Scottish Cot Death Trust – research, support, information and good practice guidelines.
Royal Hospital for Sick Children, Yorkhill, Glasgow G3 8SJ.
Tel: (041) 357 3946.

Index

Aberfan disaster, 11
abortion, spontaneous *see* miscarriage
access to child's body, 9, 73–4, 90
  preparing the body, 53, 61, 62, 90
accidental death, 8–11
  life-support withdrawal, 87
ACT, 127
adolescence:
  bereaved teenagers, 40, 109, 111
  death of adolescent, 34
  teenage suicide, 19–20, 69
AIDS, 21–2
Alder Centre, ix–xii, 3, 115, 120–2, 127
ambulance personnel, 49–51
anniversaries, 94
Association for Children with Heart
    Disorders, 18, 127
attending and listening skills, 71, 78–9,
  101

Batten's disease, 18
befriending, 101–2
bereavement theory, 24–30
  complicated grief, 28–30
  grieving for a child, 23–4, 30–44
Bowlby, John, 25, 32
British Association for Counselling, 127

cancer (childhood), 15–16
Cancer Relief Macmillan Fund, 127
carers, 24, 40–2
  support for, 75–7
chaplain (hospital), 51–2
child abuse *see* non-accidental injury
children *see* adolescence; siblings
clergy, 51–2
commemoration awards/dedications, 44
Compassionate Friends, 101, 112, 127
congenital disorders, 17–19
  incidence, 4
coroner's inquest, 9–11
coroner's post-mortem, 89–90
cot death, 6–8
  role of ambulance personnel, 51
  role of GP, 54, 55
  role of police, 64, 65
counselling for bereaved family, 102–6
counselling skills, 78–81
  general principles, 71–5

helping strategies, 79–81
  supervision, 71, 75–7
  training courses, 77–8
cultural/religious considerations, 30, 115
  mourning rituals, 42–4
  post-mortem procedures, 90
  role of clergy, 51–2
customs and rituals, 30, 42–4, 115
cystic fibrosis, 17
Cystic Fibrosis Trust, 128

disaster victims, 9, 11
doctors:
  GPs, 54–6, 88, 100
  hospital doctors, 58–60
drug misuse, 4, 21

emergency procedures, 86–8

family doctor, 54–6, 88, 100
family, support for, 99–115
  anniversaries, 94
  befriending, 101–2
  counselling, 102–6
  cultural differences, 115
  on first visiting the family, 92–4
  group meetings, 108–11, 117–20
  practical support, 99–100
  psychiatric support, 107–8
  psychotherapy, 106–7
  sibling support, 112–14
  social activities, 111
  suicide risk assessment, 94–6
family therapy, 108
family trees, 81
firefighters, 64
fostering issues, 22
Foundation for the Study of Infant
    Deaths, 101, 112, 128
friends of child:
  making a scrapbook, 80–1
  role of teacher, 69–70
funeral, 52–4, 90–2
  attendance, 91–2
  burial or cremation?, 90
  expenses, 91
  funeral directors, 52–4
  funeral rites, 43
  humanist funerals, 52

geneograms, 81
GPs, 54–6, 88, 100
grandparents, 23, 24, 36–7, 74
Grayson, Elizabeth, 65
Grief counselling and grief therapy
    (Worden, 1991), 25
grief and mourning, 23–45
group meetings (family support), 108–11
    starting a support group, 117–20

Haddington, Janet, 9
haemophiliac children, 21
health visitors, 56–8
heart deformities, 17–18
Hillsborough disaster, 11
Hindu mourning rituals, 30, 42, 43, 90
    post-mortem issues, 90
HIV and AIDS, 21–2
hospital doctors, 58–60

incidence, 3–6
    cot death, 7
    early miscarriage, 11
    neonatal death, 14
    stillbirths, 13
injury *see* accidental death; non-accidental
    injury
intensive care procedures, 86–8
Irish Sudden Infant Death Association,
    128
ISIDA, 128
Islamic mourning rituals, 42, 43, 90

Jewish mourning rituals, 43, 90

Kinder-Mourn Project, 124
Knapp, RJ, 33

Laing, RD, 108
Laura Centre, 128
laying-out procedures, 53, 61, 62, 90
legal proceedings, 9–10
life-support withdrawal, 87
listening skills, 71, 78–9
    for befriender, 101
Lockerbie disaster, 11

McKenna, Virginia, 111
Macmillan nurses, 15, 127
Malcolm Sargent Cancer Fund for
    Children, 128
Malcolm Sargent social workers, 15
malignant disease, 15–16
Marchioness sinking, 9
marital stresses/breakdown, 35–6
mementoes, 44
    album of memories, 80–1
    lock of hair, 53, 90

photographs, 44, 53, 62, 80, 90
memorial ceremonies, 44
meningitis, 16
midwives, 62–4
miscarriage, 11–12
    GPs' function, 54
    midwives' function, 62
Miscarriage Association, 128
murder, 4, 19
Muslim mourning rituals, 42, 43, 90
    post-mortem issues, 90

NABS (National Association of
    Bereavement Services), 128
NASS (National Association for Staff
    Support), 128
neonatal death, 14–15, 34
neurodegenerative disorders, 18–19
non-accidental injury, 22
    child protection social workers, 68
nurses, 60–2

Parkes, Colin Murray, 25, 32
partnership stresses/breakdown, 35–6
Peppers, LG, 33
perinatal loss, 11–15
    heart deformities, 17
    incidence, 4
    role of GP, 54
    role of midwife, 62–4
photographs:
    by police, following accidental death,
        9, 11
    of stillborn baby, 12, 62
    as treasured mementoes, 44, 53, 80, 90
police, 64–5
post-mortem examinations, 89–90
prenatal/perinatal loss, 11–15, 34
    power of parent/baby bond, 11–12,
        30, 34
professional carers, 24, 40–2
    support for, 75–7
psychiatric family support, 107–8
psychologist referrals, 107
psychotherapy, 106–7

registrars of births, marriages and death,
    66–7
religious considerations:
    mourning rituals, 42–4
    post-mortem procedures, 90
    role of clergy, 51–2
resuscitation, 87
rituals, 42–4, 80
    cultural differences, 42–3
    see also funeral
road traffic accidents, 8
    legal proceedings, 9–10

SAFTA (Support After Termination for Abnormality), 13, 129
SANDS (Stillbirth and Neonatal Death Society), 14, 63, 128
school teachers, 69–70
    suicide of school student, 20, 69
Scottish Cot Death Trust, 101, 129
seeing the body *see* viewing the body
self-help support groups, 109
siblings, 24, 37–40, 74
    attending funeral, 92
    drawing pictures, 80
    features of grief and mourning, 37–40, 113–14
    making scrapbooks, 80–1
    psychologist referrals, 107
    role of teacher, 69
    support for, 112–14
SIDS (sudden infant death syndrome), 4, 6–8
skills:
    attending and listening, 71, 78–9, 101
    counselling skills, 71–5, 78–81
social workers, 67–8
spontaneous abortion *see* miscarriage
stillbirth, 11–12, 13–14
    definition, 11
    funeral expenses, 91
    role of midwife, 62–4
Stillbirth and Neonatal Death Society (SANDS), 14, 63, 128

substance misuse, 21
sudden infant death syndrome (SIDS), 4, 6–8
suicide, 19–20
    concerns of teacher, 69
    incidence, 4
    risk assessment in bereaved parent, 94–5
supervision, 71, 75–7

TCF (Compassionate Friends), 101, 112, 127
teachers, 69–70
    suicide of school student, 20, 69
teenager *see* adolescence
termination of pregnancy, 13
    role of GP, 54
training courses, 77–8
twins:
    grief of surviving twin, 38
    neonatal loss of one twin, 14, 63

viewing the body, 9, 73–4, 90
    preparing the body, 53, 61, 62, 90
viral infections (acute), 16

Wilson, Richard, 31–2, 60
Worden, J William, 25–6, 27, 32–3
writing as therapy, 80